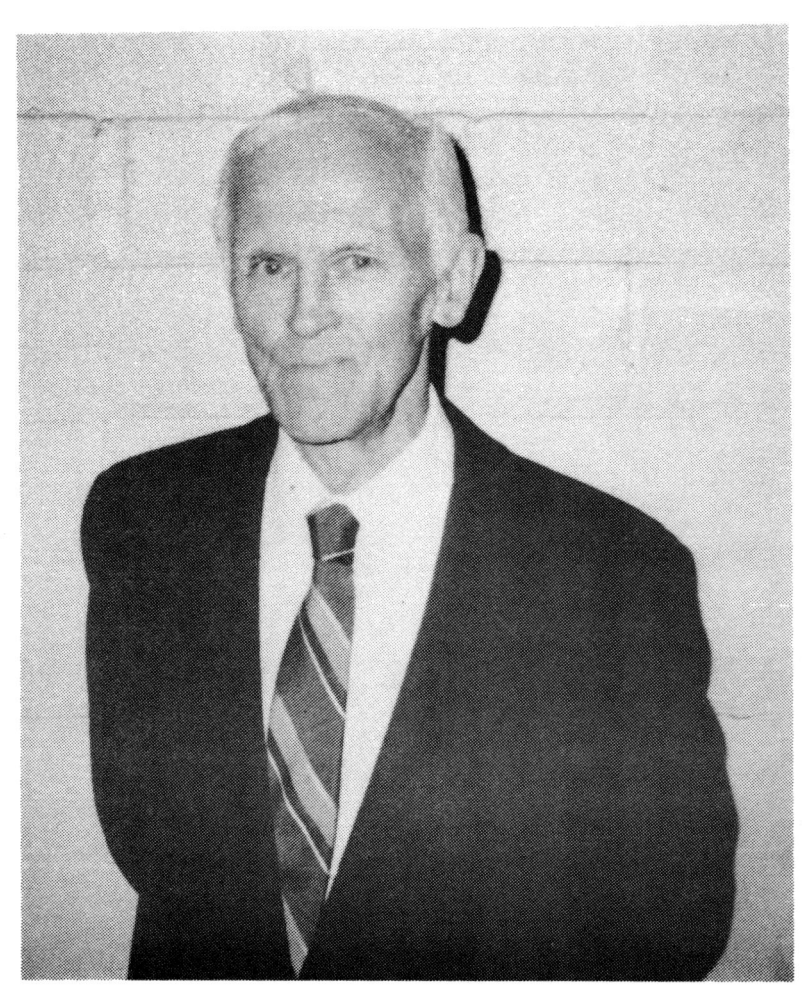

Dr. Cliff H. Robertson

THE HEALTH EXPLOSION

Cliff H. Robertson
Osteopathic Physician
Author

Caroline R. Panagos
Research Associate

Bob Darrell, Ph.D.
Editor

A. Nicholas H. Panagos
Cover Art

Robertson
11401 Herbert Rd.
Whitesville, KY 42378

All Rights Reserved

Copyright 1983 by
Dr. Cliff H. Robertson and Caroline R. Panagos

This book, *The Health Explosion,* may not be reproduced in whole or in part - except for purposes of reviews - without written permission from Dr. Cliff H. Robertson or Caroline R. Panagos. For information, write Caroline R. Panagos, Box 2375, Owensboro, Kentucky 42302.

Library of Congress Catalog Card #83-063478.

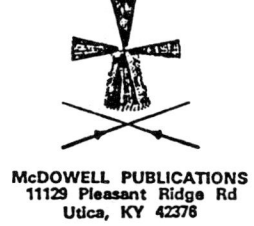

McDOWELL PUBLICATIONS
11129 Pleasant Ridge Rd
Utica, KY 42376

DEDICATIONS

To my wife, Louise, for her unending patience, understanding, support, and infinite love.

To my children, who grew up with an unconventional doctor for their father.

To my daughter, Caroline, whose enthusiasm, tireless efforts, and perserverence resulted in this book's completion.

To my granddaughter, Jennifer, who realized the need to perpetuate her grandfather's philosophy and experience while on break in Britain and who contributed a year to gathering information to launch this book.

To my patients, friends, and office and clerical staff - for their faith in me, encouragement, dedication to methods of treatment described in this book, and for their persistent requests for such a book.

To Dr. Bob Darrell, who edited and assisted in this book's publication, generously sharing his skills and wisdom.

* * * * *

I thank the following for sharing their case histories with readers of this book:

Lolita Bogdan; Dolton, Illinois

Arnold Gerhardstein Sr., father of Arnold Gerhardstein Jr.; Lamesa, California

Lawrence Hammond; Naples, Florida

Tim Hammond; Owensboro, Kentucky

Lynn Hathaway; Huntingburg, Indiana

Reverend Msgr. William B. Jarboe; Owensboro, Kentucky

Andrew Jessee; Simpsonville, South Carolina

Frances Potts; Taylors, South Carolina

Brenda Faye Wilhite, mother of Brandy Wilhite; Evansville, Indiana

Especially I express appreciation to Russelle Lear Boster for her letter concerning her son, Kirk, and to Kirk for allowing us to reprint his booklets, "The Allergy Story" and "The Allergy Kid, Part II."

ACKNOWLEDGEMENTS

I gratefully acknowledge the following for permission to reprint:

"Story of Ho-Ti" (old Chinese fable), *Introductory Physiology and Hygiene* (Indiana Edition), W. H. Conn, Ph.D. (Morristown, N.J.: Silver Burdett Company, 1904).

Picture of the Digestive Tube from *Basic Physiology and Anatomy,* Chaffee and Lytle, 4th ed. (Philadelphia: J. B. Lippincott, 1980).

Illustrations: "Topography of the Lacrimal Apparatus" and "External and Middle Ear, Opened Anteriorly (right side)," *Gray's Anatomy* ed. Charles M. Goss, 29th ed. (Philadelphia, Pa.: Lea & Febiger, 1973).

"Intestine," a definition (Digestion and Secretion), from *Webster's Third New International Dictionary* (Springfield, Mass.: Merriam-Webster, Inc., 1981).

"Colon Therapy Chart," *Colon Health: The Key to a Vibrant Life,* Norman W. Walker, D.Sc., Ph.D. (Phoenix, Arizona: O'Sullivan, Woodside & Company, 1979).

FOREWORD

Today and in the recent past, we have observed an apparent rush to approach man's physical problems on the basis of "Crisis Medicine." Naturally, this thinking and practice leads the practitioner to cover up symptoms or defects as he attempts to ease the patient's pains.

Health-care costs have risen so dramatically that one can hardly afford to be sick. The national loss in dollars, lives, and health alarms us. Lay people are becoming fed up, disillusioned by the present health-care system, and are beginning to ask why doctors do not consider human body problems from an etiological (causative) standpoint, rather than encourage patients to depend upon drugs and doctors.

When I was a student fifty years ago, a prominent minister said to me, "If you doctors were as smart as you pretend to be, you would not be such physical wrecks yourselves." His idea registered with me since my body indeed was a wreck. At that time, I suffered from many physical disorders including major sinus and colon problems.

As I studied further to seek answers, I found guidance in ancient writings and manuscripts and in modern-day health publications such as *Let's Live, Prevention Magazine, Organic Gardening and Farming, The Provoker, The N.F.A. Magazine, Acres U.S.A.,* and others. Much valuable information has also come from professional schools, seminars and conventions, and from my study of osteopathic medicine and allopathic medicine.

Probably, however, the greatest influence on my thinking and teaching has come from the philosophy of Dr. Andrew Taylor Still, the founder of Osteopathy. During my half century of practice, I have tried to follow Dr. Still's teachings.

When many disagreed with my apparently unorthodox methods, God's grace and guidance led me to understand natural healing and health, and to believe and teach my own convictions. Frequently, patients and friends have encouraged me to write a book to record, to perpetuate these techniques and philosophies for present and future generations. To readers, I offer this book, *The Health Explosion*, as a source of insight into the wonderful ways the human body God created can and does heal itself if we treat it properly.

The total plan of this book is to promote better knowledge and understanding of one's own body and to pass on to succeeding generations the application of God's laws.

CONTENTS

Dedications v
Acknowledgements vii
Foreward ix
Introduction 1
Chapter I - Diets Past and Present 7
Chapter II - Digestion and Secretion 19
Chapter III - Medicine and Disease: No Mystery 27
Chapter IV - Detoxification 37
Chapter V - Colon 39
Chapter VI - Crohn's Disease 51
Chapter VII - Ear, Nose, and Throat 57
Chapter VIII - Asthma and Emphysema 71
Chapter IX - Arthritis and Arthrosis 79
Chapter X - Cancer, Detoxification, and Nutrition 83
Chapter XI - Our Cardio-Vascular System 87
Chapter XII - Female Problems 93
Conclusion 99
Glossary 101

APPENDICES

A - The Allergy Story by The Allergy Kid 105
B - The Allergy Kid (Part II) 113

FIGURES

1 - The Digestive System 19
       Figure Repeated 39
2 - The Ptosis Support (Front view) 42
3 - The Ptosis Support (Back view) 42
4 - Dr. Robertson with Young Patient on Backswing (picture).. 43
5 - Healthy Colon 44
6 - Sick Colons 45
7 - Turbinates (Nasal cavity. Side view) 59
8 - Polyps. (Nasal cavity. Side view) 60
9 - External and Middle ear, Opened Anteriorly. (Right side) . 61
10 - Topography of the Lacrimal Apparatus 68

INTRODUCTION

Constantly, we are told that 1) America is a healthy nation, 2) we now live longer, and 3) we enjoy a fuller life than in the past. If these statements are true, why is the U.S. health status among the lowest on earth, as recorded by the United Nations statistics. The American people, as compared to people of other affluent nations, suffer from the highest percentage per capita of dental decay, heart disease, arthritis, so-called contagious diseases, and cancer. We also maintain the greatest number of medical and in-patient facilities per capita of almost any other country.

Look around you at our healthy nation. Many people today look half-baked, out of shape, swollen, bloated, bald, bland, crippled, deaf and half-dead—all signs of degeneration. I'm sure you've heard the saying, "You are what you eat." The signs, indeed, are visible. Our food and water has become so unsustaining that people resort to drugs, dope, synthetic vitamins, alcohol, additives, tobacco (the list goes on) to compensate for lack of fuel and life in their food and drink. Some scientific surveys suggest that pasteurization of our dairy products and refinement of our grains contribute to sterility and other sexual problems. We are told also that enrichment of foods with synthetic vitamins, especially grain foods, has led to a tremendous increase in heart disease in this country, a fact known for over a decade. Indiscriminate use of our microwave ovens and prescribed radiation treatments lead to destruction of various parts of our bodies, resulting perhaps in eventual total destruction.

My personal observation on the nation's state of health—recently recorded during an Osteopathic Convention (I'm sure you noticed the same conditions if you've attended a convention)—reveals that many women smoke and cough; most were flabby, out of shape; and most suffered from varicose veins. Even the few rather handsome women retained so little natural color to their faces that they plastered rouge and tinted make-up from hair lines to collar-bones.

Many doctors there appeared sickly; few appeared athletic; most wore glasses (regardless of age); and fat bellies usually accompanied worried facial expressions. When joviality occurred, it usually resulted from alcohol served with the banquet or consumed in a nearby bar.

Practically all food and drink served was sugared, highly-processed, over-cooked, and disguised with condiments to imitate flavor. Exhibits on display were dominated by drug companies, and evening speakers (supposed to entertain and inform) were sometimes slow, boring, even occasionally incoherent. No wonder doctors suffer from among the highest suicide, drug addiction, and divorce rates of all the professions.

Each hour of every day we see evidence of this decay, yet the next minute we are told how healthy we are. And it's all subtle. Ironically, as we drive along our highways, we are becoming aware of our great national health problem. Occasionally, you will see federal road signs that read, "Food, Gas, Phone, Lodging, and Hospital." When a person lives on our average American diet, those words become more than consequential; when we eat the food, we probably will develop gas, feel so terrible and tired that we need a phone to arrange lodging—if we don't become ill, indeed, so that we wind up in the hospital!

In an airport recently (and in various restaurants you, I'm sure, have observed the same), I saw a display of candy with a sign over it reading, "Help Retarded Children." Can you believe this? Have we actually sunk so far in darkness that we accept and believe that spending money to buy refined sugars helps retarded children—whose retardation these same refined products may have promoted.

Still, we are told "America is the healthiest nation on earth." Let me list more evidence of America's ill-health.

1. *Destruction of the American home as evidenced by the divorce rate, runaway children, and non-communicating family members.* When you watch "Donahue," the well-known daily television program, you are aware of the status of marriage. I have heard him interview young people who apparently do not believe in the integrity of the home unit anymore. They expound on the advantages of living together and raising their children outside of marriage. Others praise the commune in which the husband and wife are not bound legally, but rather mate with other husbands and wives as well, raise communal children, and all care for each other.

2. *Loss of morals.* We see more free love and couples living together as reported by daily news media and by reports of local law enforcement officials.

3. *Juvenile and adult delinquency.* Most of us know at least one or two youth or adults who have lived so irresponsibly that they find the law confronting them.

4. *Mental decay.* Self-evident is this problem as reflected in philosophies and policies of our business, church, and government leaders.

5. *Addiction to drugs and non-food additives.* Every day we become more aware of the terrible drug problems of our young people and their addiction to alcohol. In 1983, The National Council on Alcoholism estimated that 10 million Americans were alcoholics. I have mentioned our addiction to our diet of devitalized and nothing foods, as evidenced by our obesity, chronic illness, and fatigue.

6. *An unceasing increase in numbers of hospitals, doctors, health clinics, mental institutions, and nursing homes.* And why not? It is accepted and sociable to be ill or to have an operation. I am confident that most of you know a friend or acquaintance who cannot wait to corner you to tell you of his/her latest visit to the doctor or most recent operation. We have become

Introduction

more accustomed to ill-health than to good health. Through our insurance and government subsidy programs, we not only are encouraged to be sick, but also we are paid well to be ill. And costs climb daily. The technology necessary to analyze a physical problem is overwhelming. Ten years ago, it cost $75,000.00 to die of cancer; the American Cancer Society today has revised this amount to an inestimable figure.

Today, a person surviving a heart attack will have to shell out anywhere from $10,000.00 to $50,000.00. An acquaintance recently accumulated bills in excess of $75,000.00 in 30 days for a case of severe burns. Even the nation-wide cost of the common cold for one year, is unbelievable, when you consider medical expenses, drugs, and loss of work hours industry must absorb.

How long can this nation afford these escalations? How much longer can the human body tolerate this abuse without becoming extinct?

Personally, I like to think that we are waking up, wising up, wanting better lives, willing to act to build better health conditions. Almost any popular publication issued today will carry at least one article relating to health, diet, or the relationship of one to the other.

During the past few years, I have recognized a promising change in America's sense of its health. The public no longer is content with the sloppy, complacent TV lounger, but now respects the fit and shapely joggers and strives to emulate them.

This change partially resulted from reevaluation of health standards brought about by research and studies done by both governmental and private organizations. Some of these studies linked diet, exercise (rather lack of it), toxins and pollutants, and so forth to cancer and heart disease. This philosophy—that diet directly affects health—long had been advocated by many noted nutritionists the world over, and this idea prompted many studies. Back in the 30's and 40's and 50's, the health trend in California helped to begin this movement, which now spreads throughout our nation.

Today—indeed, as you read these words—all walks of life obtain nutrition messages from the media, whether it be dog food, with perhaps fewer calories and more bone meal, or people food, with perhaps additional vitamins and minerals. And the population now searches for better information and answers.

As I travel about our country, speaking frequently to schools, colleges, church groups, and conventions—both professional and non-professional—I have become aware of the disgust at some practices we doctors today are guilty of. Even though it cuts deeply into my personal and professional feelings, I can understand how these people are justified in their criticisms.

The most common complaint I hear is that "You doctors never do anything constructive to help us get and stay well. You only make us more dependent on doctors and medicines." One purpose of this book is to teach readers how they can depend less on doctors. Medicine was meant to prevent and alleviate disease, not to create a chronic dependence on physicians.

Today's practice of medicine has resulted largely from a treatment of and obliterating of disease symptoms, rather than from promoting good health.

In the first place, a physician is by tradition supposedly a teacher. Why have we strayed from this divine, high-level of instructing others? I wish to teach readers that they can live long and healthy lives *free from fears of dreaded diseases.*

Much of my knowledge and information I obtained by studying a variety of written sources. Many helpful books pertaining to health and nutrition await you in most bookstores. I have learned much and still am learning from many of these books, written by both professional and non-professional people.

From these studies and from my travels, I find much evidence that people can practice self-healing successfully, and I notice a growing trend in this practice today. These people, experimenting with self-healing, obtain most information from their friends and acquaintances and from studying these books. As a matter of fact, from studying practically disease-free nationalities of various geographical areas, and from realizing that these areas actually do exist, I learned to investigate and to try some alternative healing practices. This approach I continue to do, and I am learning that methods used by these healthy disease-free peoples will work on anybody—if we but apply them, remembering their natural law basis. But we must study and understand these natural laws.

I attended school to become an osteopathic physician, learning laws to guide me in healing the sick, but I left school with little knowledge of health. After graduation, and in my twenties, I became so sick with asthma, colitis, clogged sinuses, and other ailments that I then began my search for cures, better methods of cure than I had learned while in college. This search has brought me to this day and this book.

I am writing to demonstrate to readers that natural healing is not only alive and well, but also that it still succeeds. The human body is a magnificent creature, with great healing power and does possess the ability to rebuild totally under correct conditions every seven years. And the "practice of medicine" is the vehicle by which this rebuilding occurs.

But today's interpretation of *medicine* digresses far from the original idea conventionally defined as "the science and art of dealing with the prevention, cure, or alleviation of disease," and "in a narrower sense, that part of the science and art of restoring and preserving health."

Since we are supposed to practice medicine, we should practice with our current knowledge, using God's laws as we uncover them, not forgetting the natural laws used in healing by man from the beginning of recorded history

Introduction

and eliminating those practices tried and proven unsuccessful. We must grow constantly in our learning as we daily apply these principles of healing to seek the truth, ever-cautious to prevent pride and ego from destroying our *true* purpose of healing and helping mankind.

At our clinic, we begin treatment of any physical problem by trying to discover its cause. Then, we proceed to eliminate or correct that cause. In my practice, cause is the ultimate key to unlocking the door to recovery. This procedure I have applied for almost a half century. Let me illustrate what I have said.

As we pull into our driveway after a long, tiring trip, we notice our house on fire. No doubt, in our mind a problem exists. We face several alternatives. It would be hard to ignore that the house is on fire because we feel heat and see flames rising. The sensible thing to do would be to call the fire department to douse the flame. And after the fire was extinguished, firemen would determine the fire's cause because that is the fireman's normal course of action—his job.

There exists another alternative, stupid as it may sound. You could choose to ignore that the house is on fire. We could erect a huge masonite screen so we could neither see the flames nor feel the heat. The fire would remain, but for awhile we would remain unaware of it. Smoke would soon rise from behind the screen, and we would again be aware of a problem. Now, had we called the fire department and it had doused the fire, the smoke would soon subside. If, however, we still choose to ignore the fire, we could throw a huge tarpaulin over the house and fire. The smoke would still continue to accumulate, but we could ignore that, too.

Soon, we would begin to notice a strong stench in the air. Had we called the fire department, this stench, too, soon would go away. But had we followed our second alternative, we could simply place a clothespin on our noses and refuse to smell.

An amusing supposition, you say. But isn't this approach our procedure regarding pain? Aware that something is causing pain, why do we reach for a pain killer rather than attempt to locate the pain's cause?

When the alchemist first produced pain-killing drugs, men and women began drifting from the original purpose of medication—the science and art dealing with prevention, cure, or alleviation of disease. After my forty-eight years of practice, I am more convinced now than ever before that the practice of modern medicine is retrogressing to the practices of the Middle Ages, a period of time we don't hear too much about in medicine today.

William Dufty's chapter "How We Got Here From There" in his book, *Sugar Blues*, explains how practices of medicine evolved from the natural healers of old to today's highly technological medical institutions. *Sugar Blues* is an interesting, informative book (published by Warner Books), and you can find it in most natural food stores. Mr. Dufty goes into detail on the history of healing and explains many different remedies. Even today, we are still experimenting with a multitude of new and old methods, practicing those that bring good results and eliminating—we hope—those producing adverse effects.

This book results from my years of practice—accumulating much evidence through experience and clinical research, incorporating those methods with good results, and rejecting others less desirable.

Chapter I

DIETS PAST AND PRESENT

Before modern civilization, food was eaten almost as soon as it left its life source. Human beings lived on fruits, berries, nuts, grains, roots, and vegetation (usually in its raw state). Wild game was the meat, requiring vigorous chewing; anything cooked probably was cooked minimally. How does your table compare with this apparently early practice in food selection and preparation?

A VISIT TO OUR SUPERMARKET

Most Americans buy their food from local supermarkets, which generally organize their foods in a particular fashion.

Fresh Foods. Usually, the large chains position fresh foods on either side of the first aisle. Except in an unusually large store in an unusually large city, fresh raw foods and root foods will utilize only two aisles of the market. Within these two aisles, you find fruits; nuts; red, yellow, and green vegetables; sprouts (if you're lucky); and root crops such as potatoes and onions. Even then, however, it will be almost impossible to find one item of these beautiful specimens not sprayed with a chemical in the field, fumigated in storage to keep off bugs, or microwaved or radiated to prevent spoilage.

Other Foods and Meats. Other food aisles contain grains and grain products; canned, frozen, or packaged fruits, juices, and vegetables; and meats. Meats come from animals fed hormones and chemically-treated grains; fruits, as a whole, will be loaded with sugars; vegetables have been highly processed; rice is polished; and pastas are derived from refined grains. All of these, you can be almost certain, were treated chemically during their growing-season.

Dairy Products. At the dairy bar, if you read labels on cheeses, cheese foods, and milk products, you'll encounter these terms: pasteurized, homogenized, ultra-pasteurized, sugar, corn syrup, mono- and diglycerides, artificial flavor, carrageenan, whipping gas, nitrous oxide, and the list goes on and on and on referring to processes, artificial additives, even dyes.

Breads. Next, if you check your market's bread bin, you might ask yourself, "Can I find whole wheat or whole grain bread?" Don't select loaves announcing whole wheat, cracked wheat, or rye because they may only carry a trace of that specific grain. See if you can find the one that reads one-hundred-percent whole wheat. Don't be too surprised, then, when you notice all the additives listed for that loaf.

Now you may want to ask yourself "Has our conception of good health changed throughout history?" A second question occurs: Indeed, don't we relate proper diet and good health?

VITAMINS AND MINERALS

Apparently, today we are as much or more concerned with vitamin and mineral supplements than with actual diet. We need to ask this question: "Are supplements really necessary?" I am convinced that they constitute an *immediate,* necessary answer to our current nutrition dilemma, (and I depend upon them to some extent in my practice). Although the greatest miracle today is the amazing degree of health we enjoy in spite of the atrocious environmental insults we are subjected to daily, demands on our bodies to overcome these insults are greater than ever before. Bodies now nourished by depleted soils (soils all over our world depleted of nutritive ingredients) consuming depleted diets need maximum nutrition offered in supplements to overcome these deficiencies and other environmental insults.

Supplements, however, we should use only with advice and expert assistance—a doctor or qualified nutritionist. Carefully selected reading, however, not only will help you increase your awareness of how to establish good diet practices—including food selection and preparation—but also increase your awareness of benefits and limitations regarding vitamins and mineral supplements. You can locate many good books on health and nutrition at natural food stores, which will help to educate you on different vitamins and minerals.

Our society fails to stress adequately that *minerals* form the foundation of the body's building stones. In that respect, *proportional amounts* of *all* nutritive elements are of the utmost importance, and not the amount of each individual mineral itself. We must remain cautious and choose nutritive supplements wisely.

These supplements should be investigated thoroughly. A good supplement should be all natural: contain no refined sugars, artificial, or synthetic additives; include *no* filler; and they should derive directly from some living plant or animal.

Beware of merely analytical advice about the composition of a vitamin, mineral, or food. Remember, not only is analysis of the particular food or element valuable but also important is the body's reaction to that element. The greatest laboratory in the world is your own body: Watch it and listen to it.

COMMENTS ON MINERALS

I want to share with you my observations on a few nutritive elements.

Calcium. Calcium builds red blood. Researchers tell us that only three percent of Americans possess sufficient calcium. A calcium shortage apparently causes anxiety. Calcium is a balancer; it cannot work without vitamins A, C, D, and phosphorus, and cannot be assimilated without vitamin F. A mother's milk, for example, needs calcium, phosphorus, and manganese, which can be obtained through sea vegetation such as kelp, greens, and many edible weeds found in the lawn and garden. These can be eaten raw or steamed, and include dandelion, lamb's-quarter, wild violet, wild garlic and onions, chick weed, buckhorn, sorrell, plantain, borage, valerian, polk weed, wild mustard, milkweed, thistle, tender young sassafras leaves, and many others. These greens possess high mineral content. Another good source of calcium is ground whole beef bone which, I might add, contains all the minerals of the body. This is highly assimilable. A good way to make your own bone marrow supplement is to cut long bones in pieces, short enough to dig the bone marrow out. This marrow then can be mixed with herbs and other tasty raw foods.

Calcium is the necessary element in forming the cement which holds our body cells together.

Iodine. According to estimates, an average body contains twenty-five milligrams of iodine. Iodine is a trace mineral and a part of thyroxin. Thyroxin is a hormone secreted by the thyroid gland, which enters every cell of the body for the purpose of controlling the rate at which the cell uses oxygen. When a person eats natural poison-free foods, with a liberal supply of seaweed, it is difficult to consume too much iodine.

Iron. Iron is a trace mineral found in every cell of all living things, both plant and animal. Most iron in the human body is a component of hemoglobin (an oxygen-carrying protein of the red blood cells) and myoglobin (an oxygen-carrying protein of the muscle cells). Their function is to carry and release oxygen. Iron deficiency can cause anemia, indicated by fatigue, weakness, apathy, even headaches. Iron also works with an enzyme which helps to create neurotransmitters — substances that carry messages from one nerve cell to another. Decreased attentiveness, lower-than-usual IQ, and hyperactivity also can indicate iron deficiency. Good sources to ensure an adequate supply of iron are dark greens, legumes, whole grains, and dried fruits such as apricots, raisins, peaches, and prunes. Iron can never be assimilated without a trace of copper. Both iron and copper are found in a most perfect form in sea vegetation.

Potassium. Potassium contributes directly to appropriate strength of the body and brain. Even a slight deficiency of potassium can lead to slow growth. Lack of potassium can cause certain types of insanity and frequently can cause birth defects. One of the best sources of potassium is apple cider vinegar or honey in the comb. Other food sources include potatoes, dried fruits, bananas, and orange juice.

Zinc. Though true that the body needs only a trace of zinc, that trace is important especially for healing purposes. Only in recent years have we discovered that zinc is as important as protein in the normal growth process and maintenance of body tissue. An infant's liver contains twice as much zinc as an adult's. Prime sources of zinc in animal foods are oysters, herring, egg yolks, and milk; whole grains, sea vegetation, and alfalfa are the richest among plant foods.

ECOLOGY-BASED FOODS

Foods should be based ecologically. As much as possible, foods comprising the greater portion of our diet should grow in the area we live in. When we begin to eat food imported from other climatic regions, we lose our adaptability to our environment. This imbalance often leads to sickness, manifested in either our bodies or minds, or both. This result is especially true where tropical or semi-tropical products are consumed in temperate climates. Also, serious illness can result from overconsumption of heavy animal food by people in a warmer climate since this type of food is more suited to cold regions. Ideally, food should be chosen from within a 3-500 mile radius of our homes; however, if not possible, the next best choice of foods would be from areas with climates similar to ours.

Since most all areas of our country grow grains, and we all consume some type of grain, let's next examine them.

WHOLE GRAINS

Today, poison-free whole grains are so readily available that we see no excuse for not using them exclusively. In the early days of my practice in Owensboro, Kentucky, these grains were not available. Since I strongly desired to see my patients eat whole-grain bread, I found a mill twenty miles away that would grind and bag one-hundred-percent whole wheat flour and whole corn meal. Then, I transported this flour in the trunk of my car and left it with patients as I made house-calls. Before long, I discovered that another local source, the Anglo-American Meal Company, was grinding wonderful whole-grain flour. Occasionally, when this company had some flour to spare, it let us know. With these contacts, a miller friend and I supplied local supermarkets and restaurants. Some Saturdays, we set up displays in supermarkets, where someone demonstrated how to use whole grain and corn meal and served small samples of bread. When a local bakery began succeeding at baking and selling our whole grain breads, I realized public users of whole grains would buy these products if available.

Today, it is your and my responsibility to demand—to ensure—that safe bread is available to the American public. Dr. Joe Nichols, noted Texas physician and author of the book, *Please Doctor, Do Something*, has stated, "What America needs badly is a good loaf of bread."

The staff of life has become the club of death. The time has come for us to wake up and to quit taking the life out of our foundation foods. Our millers are removing much of the vitamin and mineral content from whole grain, and they blame this act on public demand. Then, they replace these elements with four synthetic minerals—something totally foreign to human beings. You can write the United States Printing Office for a tract on this

Diets Past and Present

country's milling process to see what actually happens to whole grain when processed. The removed portions of the grain are fed to animals. These animals don't have to live in heated and air-conditioned homes. Along with the synthetic minerals, baked into the bread, the miller also includes preservatives and other additives. A nationally-known chemist declared that additives in our bread and the lack of germ and bran rank as the number one cause of heart disease in Americans today. If you read the history of bread in America, you will find that the incidence of heart disease increased rapidly following the addition of synthetic iron to American flour.

Wheat. But there is more to a fine loaf of bread than its source. Flour should be ground immediately preceding the baking process and will retain more life if ground by a steel burr rather than a stone burr. This fresh milling is necessary to prevent flour oils from oxidizing. When grain oils remain exposed to the air for many hours, they rapidly deteriorate and become toxins. These toxins created by rancidity and the lack of the body's ability to digest starch then can cause an accumulation of heavy mucous in the head and sinuses, eventually harming the body's system. This deterioration leads to development of degenerative diseases—especially arthritis, heart disease, and collections of cholesterol deposits on inside walls of arteries.

Therefore, you must strive for freshly ground whole grains, preferably organically grown, in your bread—with ample bulk and fiber. If desired, the sweetener should be sorghum or honey, and the oil should be a good, cold-pressed, fresh vegetable oil (non-chemically treated).

Corn. A good wheat bread substitute is corn bread. I recommend highly live corn, grown from open pollinated seed. Indians certainly fared well on it. To enjoy the delicacy of corn, you should use it first in whole grain form. You can sprout it and eat both sprout and grain. If you choose not to consume it this way, you can grind it into meal. If you prefer to buy your corn meal, ensure that it has not been refined or degerminated, is ground fresh, and has been refrigerated. Likewise, when you bring this flour home and are through using it from the bag, place it in the refrigerator. Corn is delicious when ground and steamed as a mush for breakfast or served with a meal. A coarser grind, such as grits, is even better as a cereal. Eaten this way, however, grits require at least thirty chews to masticate it completely. If more flavor is desired, you may add honey or maple syrup.

Grains for Hot Cereals. Wheat, rye, and barley create excellent body-building hot cereals. These grains you prepare either by soaking the grain till it swells and then heating it in hot water or by bringing the water to a boil, pouring in the grain, and removing it from the burner to swell.

Processed Cereals. Don't be fooled into thinking that because a food is called a cereal and derives from natural grains, that it is necessarily a wholesome body-building food. In fact, some cereals are the exact opposite. I refer to most ordinary packaged dry cereals found on your grocery shelf. Most of these cereals contain added sugar, have been subjected to high heat processing, have synthetics added as substitutes for natural ingredients, have been fumigated with chemicals while in storage as grains, have been stored in the boxes for a period of time which allows grain oils to deteriorate, and have been refined and devitalized by refining processes.

I found it sadly amusing to hear that one of our eastern universities did some research on commercially-packaged cereals. They fed one test group of animals contents of the cereal carton, cereal only; and a second test group were fed cartons only. The result, as I'm sure you guessed, was that animals fed the cartons outlived animals fed the cereal. This finding was demonstrated further to me when I read of Dr. Joe Nichols' account (in *Please Doctor, Do Something*); he stored a box of packaged cereal in his garage for more than a year, and none of it was bothered by insects or animals.

Do we actually want foods animals won't touch? The grocer says that he must supply what the public demands. Are we still demanding these foods—these foods full of additives and sugars?

SUGAR

SUGAR AND HISTORY

In 1939, during World War II, Hitler's armies marched into Vienna, and they confiscated all the sugar they could find. Soon after, heart disease in Austria decreased tremendously. At the same time, the ulcer rate in the German army increased greatly. Germans on the Russian front, however, eating the same food as the Russians, had an almost total decrease in stomach ulcers. After Hitler's armies removed the sugar from Holland, that country's cancer rate decreased more than fifty percent during the four years of occupation.

Some writers on ancient history suggest that the fall of the Roman Empire resulted largely from the use of sugar. According to ancient records, Turks or their predecessors began refining sugar. Today, it is an established fact that habitual use of refined sugars creates a desire for alcohol and other stimulants. In his book, *Vermont Folk Medicine*, Dr. Jarvis tells how he actually changed alcoholics into non-alcoholics by using honey. He fed alcoholics quantities of pure honey until it would cause them to dislike the taste of alcohol.

We are a nation of sugar-holics. Look in your pantry and try to find one can or box that does not contain a sugar-added food. You may find a few canned vegetables without processed sugars, but you will be surprised how many products containing added sugar you do find.

SUGAR'S HARMFUL EFFECTS

Well, you say, "What's wrong with a little sugar, anyway?" For a start, you must read *Sugar Blues* by William Dufty. It alone should make you a sugar teetotaler.

Diets Past and Present

Each day we learn more about sugar's harmful effects. Athletes develop cramps from it; statistics indicate that sugar, not fat, is a major cause of heart trouble; most any teenager thinks that sugar causes acne; through research, psychologists explain that sugar causes hyperactive children; dentists blame it for dental cavities; and physiologists explain how sugar arrests secretion of stomach gastric juices and causes body decalcification by neutralizing calcium in the blood (an immediate condition).

How do we wean ourselves from sugar? History demonstrates that some sweeteners are safe for life. The two safest sweets are raw honey and pure date sugar. The best raw honey should be unheated, untreated, and in the comb. A diabetic, in some cases, can eat raw honey because it supposedly contains insulin. Incidentally, another good source of insulin is the Jerusalem Artichoke, also called the Sunchoke. We must recognize that sugar and honey differ from each other; further, this difference lies in the body's action on or reaction to any food, including sugar.

HONEY

I have used much honey in my seventy-year lifetime, mostly raw honey in the comb. For many of my earlier years, I had a heart murmur, or heart leak, discovered in my college days when I was told that it was caused by rheumatic fever. Nonetheless, I now have, and have had for some years, a strong heart muscle and no evidence of the leak or murmur. I do not imply that honey by itself caused regeneration of my heart, since many other factors may appertain. For example, I developed vigorous exercise programs for myself, including boxing, and I walked everywhere since I had no car. And lucky enough to live in the country, we had access to nearly perfect food. But I am convinced that the honey did play an important role in my recovery. Each year, especially in the major motel-chain restaurants, I notice an increasing availability of honey. Today, we can find honey in almost any restaurant, and some of them even serve raw sugar.

Though raw sugar represents improvement over old refined white sugar, it still has been heated and refined enough to cause arthritis or arthrosis. Any natural sugar usually Levo Rotatory changes when heated to Dextro Rotatory. We know these sugars change—from a light test showing the direction of light rays through a prism. If the light deflects to the left, the sugar is Levo Rotatory; and if the light deflects to the right, it is Dextro Rotatory. Dextro Rotatory sugars are inclined to and do decalcify the body and are known to be toxic to any animal. Honey, however, is a pure, natural food taken directly from the bees that created it. It contains iodine, iron, calcium, phophorus, and multiple vitamins. *It is perfectly balanced and easily digested* and, in my experience, always can be used in place of sugar.

FATS AND OILS

Since I apparently am discussing ingredients related to baked products, let me briefly mention fats and oils. As I said earlier, a good oil for the bread dough should be a fresh, cold-pressed vegetable oil. Never use mineral oil as a food since it is dead and will coat the intestinal wall and adhere to it. If you want to use butter, raw and unsalted, cow, goat, or sheep butter would be the better choice. Do not use any hydrogenated butter since hydrogenation changes the nature of fat, causing cholesterol to adhere to inner walls of arteries. Lecithin is the anticholesterol that always occurs in nature to keep cholesterol in solution. It is an antidote for high density lipo-proteins. Thirty percent of the dry matter of the brain is lecithin. Interestingly, lecithin is mixed into chocolate to make it metabolize. But to minimize additional cholesterol, I consider it much safer to use a vegetable oil. Probably the best choices are sesame oil, olive oil, and sunflower oil. Oils are preferred to animal fats because oils derive from vegetable sources.

VEGETABLE JUICES

Before finishing this chapter, I should mention vegetable juices. I have enjoyed remarkable results using wheat grass juice, carrot juice, and other vegetable and fruit juices for treatment of everything from skin ailments to tumors.

In our greenhouse (attached to our clinic), we grow wheat grasses for juice, plus other vegetables in the winter season. Because the greenhouse is near, we can pick fresh vegetables and grasses for juices for our patients. Rapid absorption of wheat grass juice into the blood is evidenced by flushed cheeks immediately after consumption. I remember a lady patient from Pennsylvania who was leaving the clinic and going home for Christmas several years ago. She had such colorful lips that I was prompted to ask her if she might be wearing lipstick, which I had never seen her wear. She assured me that she did not use lipstick and the color was her own. During her two-week stay here, she consumed no cooked foods. Her diet during this period included fresh carrot and wheat grass juices four times a day, along with fresh and dried organically-grown fruits and raw vegetable salads.

NURSING MOTHERS AND SPECIAL DIETS

Patients ask, "Does a nursing mother need a special diet, and how long can she adequately nurse her child?"

If a nursing mother's diet contains most of the items described below, she need not stop nursing her child before the child becomes two or three years old. Diet during that nursing period should include the following:

1. Fresh, poison-free, raw foods constituting at least ninety percent of the mother's total diet. In winter when she can't obtain fresh vegetables, she can always buy fresh seeds for sprouting. A good source is her natural food store, where she can find organically-grown or biologically-grown seeds for sprouting.

Diets Past and Present

2. Grains may be eaten if freshly ground and barely cooked at a low temperature.

3. Water must be chemically free and pure. Most city water supplies have at least a minimum of 27 added chemicals.

4. Meat is not necessary in the diet to make good milk. If the mother desires meat, meat should be from animals not treated with antibiotics or other drugs and not fed hormones. Meat should be cooked at a low temperature and most always eaten rare. More preferable would be ocean fish or fish from northern streams and lakes where pollution fallout is low. Better still, as a substitute for meat, raw nuts as well as edible seeds are much more desirable.

5. In the ten-percent category of cooked foods, some good suggestions are potatoes baked in the jacket, baked root vegetables, fresh salad greens, and other fresh vegetables lightly steamed.

If the mother desires bread, it should be baked, preferably of freshly-ground one-hundred-percent whole rye or wheat, open pollinated corn, millet, flax, or sesame seed.

Also, we recommend that the nursing mother eat liberally of honey in the comb, especially Tupelo honey, high in Levulose. Adequate amounts of sea plants in her diet, either in whole form or tablets, are also valuable to her milk. If the mother desires juices, it is much better to prepare them fresh, using only one or two vegetables juiced together. Fruit juices, with citrus juice as the lesser part, may be used if unsweetened.

It is important for the new-born baby to begin nursing almost immediately after birth to gain colostrum benefits. As stated in the chapter on "Colon," this colostrum in mother's milk is a natural mobilizer (laxative) for the new life. It contains the natural flora necessary for the colon, the foundation for the child's future health and happiness; and it begins the immune system. Babies not fortunate enough to receive their mother's milk but raised on artificial formulas usually begin their earliest days with constipation problems, which continue throughout life. Today, I see teenagers suffering with Crohn's Disease, partially resulting from absence of colostrum during their infancy. Their bowel has degenerated already to such a serious state that it would seem impossible for the colon to ever recover. We are discovering, however, that, in spite of this prevailing condition, if the patient will cooperate in a regenerative program, the colon can and does return to relative normality. (Additional discussion of Crohn's Disease occurs in the chapter on this subject.)

If mothers, for one reason or another, have babies or children who have not received natural colostrum, what can these mothers do about this deficiency? Today, colostrum from cow's milk is being marketed. A friend in Atlanta, Georgia, owns and operates one of the largest raw milk dairies in America and produces colostrum for the American market. Though this product remains inferior to the mother's colostrum, it is imperative that babies who start out on artificial milk containing no colostrum, receive it or a similar product. The next alternative is to place the baby on fresh raw vegetable juice as early as possible,—at first diluting with water until the baby's stool is stablized. If diarrhea occurs, add more water; if stool is too light, add less water and add a little honey.

DIET FOR CHILDREN AFTER NURSING

The food transition to solids from breast milk should begin with raw fruits. Blend these without any seasoning, except where honey may be needed. After starting the child on blended raw fruits and after the child's bowel movements are beginning to be well-formed, the child should receive small amounts of blended raw vegetables. If you do not have a blender, these vegetables may be ground through a food chopper. Also, it would benefit the child to add a little seaweed to the vegetable. If the child's bowels are too loose on raw foods, these foods may be steamed and then blended or chopped.

As the child begins to toothe, and has some tooth-chewing surfaces, the child may begin to eat whole raw foods. When the child begins to eat at the table with the family, it is best to serve raw foods first. That is, salad should be eaten first and slowly. Gradually, as more teeth develop, and the child can chew well, then he or she may eat the family diet, eliminating milk products entirely. Let me stress here that in consuming a raw meal, a person should allow nearly one hour to masticate thoroughly the food, and the same is more necessarily true for a meal including cooked food.

Generally, one should plan the child's raw diet in this order:

1. Breakfast should consist of fruit, berries, or melon. Fresh whole grain cereals may be substituted.
2. The noon meal should consist of vegetables. If vegetables do not satisfy totally the appetite, then raw nuts may be added.
3. The evening meal, likewise, should consist of fruits or occasionally raw vegetables.

Drink little with a meal. Small amounts of fluid may be sipped, but too much liquid will dilute the stomach juices and hinder proper digestion.

Your growing children can live and grow extremely well on a raw diet. After nearly fifty years of practice, during which time I was taught that we must eat hot-cooked meals, I have seen this raw diet work—first, to my surprise—over and over and over again. Not only will this diet produce a beautifully dispositioned and healthy child, but also it can and does heal a sick one.

I have a pair of patients, twins, who had or have Recklinghausen's Neurofibromatosis. Portions of an article printed in their home-town newspaper shortly after they began their recovery appear below:

HARTFORD - Amy and Ann Faust are like most eight-year-old twins. They do a lot of things together. They chase after their rambunctious wirehair fox terrier, Cuddles. They play doctor, pretending to take the blood pressure and temperature of an unsuspecting visitor.

Amy and Ann are also a little different. At least, they eat a little differently: they eat organic apples by the bushel, drink carrot juice by the gallon but can rarely have common foods like baked potatoes.

The twins aren't on fad diets. They are two of the approximately 100,000 people in the U.S. who have Von Recklinghausen's Neurofibromatosis, a hereditary disease affecting the nervous system, muscles, bones, and skin, for which medical doctors told Ray and Arlene Faust there is no cure.

The Fausts took the twins to what seemed to Mrs. Faust like "a different doctor every day." The doctors agreed there is no cure.

Friends recommended Robertson, an Owensboro, Kentucky, osteopath who treats patients with a strict organic diet.

Mrs. Faust said she believes the way Robertson "kneads them like dough" on their week-long semi-annual trips to Robertson's Kentucky clinic and the natural foods diet has reduced the tumors on the girls' bodies. Their color is back; their coordination is better, she said.

Today, the girls, now 13, are active and normal, healthy growing young ladies.

As I deal with specific diseases, I will mention again diets preferable to benefit those specific conditions. Since we have our thoughts on diet, let's next consider digestion.

Chapter II

DIGESTION AND SECRETION

Essentially a chemical process, digestion utilizes certain body juices to convert nutritive material to forms the body can absorb. This activity occurs through decomposing and dissolving secretions containing enzymes, assisted by the body's mechanical action. In higher animals, it begins with the saliva's action and continues as food passes through the greater part of the alimentary canal, acted upon by gastric, liver, pancreatic, and intestinal juices. Figure 1 presents The Human Digestive System.

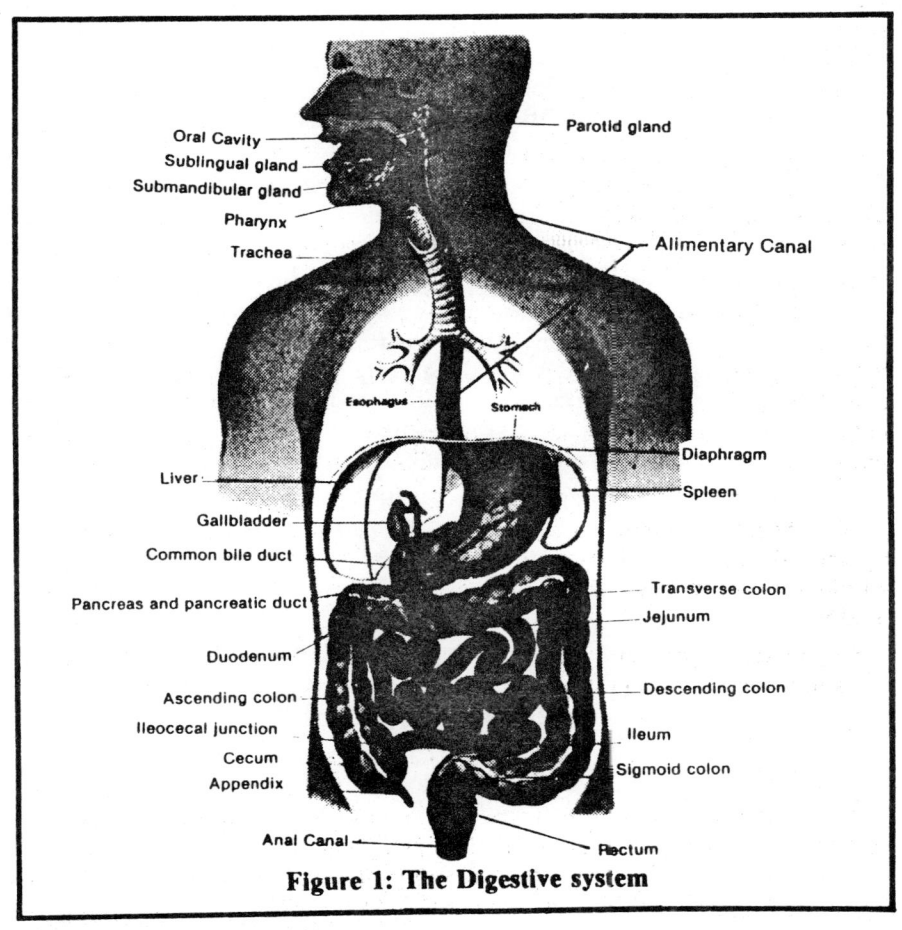

Figure 1: The Digestive system

As food reaches the stomach, digestion continues to occur. Observing our commercialization of indigestion, however, a visitor from another planet might think that what occurs normally is *indigestion*. A day does not pass without a digestive aid being advertised on radio or television. At cashier counters of most restaurants and checkout counters of grocery stores, you will find digestive aids—not a good advertisement for restaurants or grocery stores. In most cases, these aids add to the problem of digestion, by creating a more *alkaline* stomach condition when actually the stomach cries for more *acid*.

When food is chewed in the mouth, the stomach produces an appetite juice, the forerunner of other digestive juices, mainly pepsin, HCL (hydrochloric acid), and gastric lipase. If there is insufficient secretion of HCL, then the stomach fails to produce pepsin, absolutely essential for protein digestion. Lime in our water neutralizes the stomach's acidity and disturbs HCL production. If there is insufficient acid, digestion is impaired in the stomach, and the stomach will refuse to open at the distal end, where food enters the small intestine. Food then will stay in the stomach longer than intended, which helps stimulate formation of stomach gas.

On the other hand, when stomach acidity stands at the absolutely necessary amount, the end of the stomach (or pylorus) automatically opens, letting prepared stomach food enter the small intestine, ready for the next stage.

As this intestinal content moves along with the aid of liver and pancreatic secretions, the small intestine secretions come into play to help continue the digestive process. Digestion moves right along throughout the small intestine, and as the food components are prepared properly, they are collected or absorbed through the small intestine wall by means of minute villae, small teat-like projections extending from the wall into the intestine - actually shaped more like coral antennae.

The absorbed constituents (now food for the body) then are transported by body fluids to each body cell. An amazing thing about this process is that within the blood both food and toxins are carried side by side without mixing.

So you see, digestion occurs in several stages. I like to list them like this: ingestion, secretion, digestion, absorption, transportation, and assimilation.

INGESTION

Think of ingestion as an introduction of food to the digestive system through the act of eating. Generally, dictionaries indicate that ingestion means pouring, putting food into the stomach, etc. I am asked, "I eat; what should I not eat?" "What foods are good for me, and what foods will hurt me?"

These questions always remind me of the story about the fellow, troubled about his arm hurting, who went to see his doctor. The man asked the

Digestion and Secretion

doctor, "Doctor, every time I raise my arm over my shoulder like this, it hurts. What should I do?" The doctor replied, "Well, don't raise your arm over your shoulder like that."

Seriously speaking, however, things we do and foods we eat cause this degeneration and disease plaguing our world today. Listen to your body! If eating certain foods causes pain, don't eat those foods. When your stomach informs you it is full, quit eating. When thirsty, drink pure fluids. When hungry, eat only to satisfy that hunger.

Most people don't realize that nature designed eating to be done in a specific, precise manner. We have become too busy, too preoccupied with productivity, too hurried, too much creatures of habit to allow eating its proper attention.

The ceremony of eating—characteristic of many nations—is based on more than tradition or ceremony. Recent experiments in Japan, reported in a current science magazine, definitely prove that people who take much time to eat during a meal live longer, healthier lives. So, slow down and think about eating. These rules will lead to better digestion:

1. A person should never eat unless hungry. In our civilized system, we constantly are prodded to eat, as we are exposed constantly to food. Almost any commercial establishment sells some form of food.

2. Do not be addicted to the bad habit of eating a certain number of prescribed meals daily. If you notice how animals eat, you will see that they eat smaller quantities and eat more frequently than man. Naturally, you may be hungry more often when you live on a diet of whole raw foods such as the animal's diet of nuts, seeds, fruits, raw vegetables, and berries. Probably nature planned for us to be nibblers.

3. Take ample time to chew, since chewing slowly helps food to mix better with the saliva that begins food breakdown; food was designed to be liquified in the mouth as needed in the stomach. Thorough chewing with the teeth in a good jaw is essential to food digestion. Ensure that your saliva is running and thoroughly mixed with foods before you swallow. Human beings fail to chew food long enough. Each bite should be chewed thirty times, with conscious counting, until this becomes habit. As you take longer to eat, you will find you do not need to eat as much. You also may discover that you won't eat as much because you won't have the time. Let me note here that many headaches are caused by careless and insufficient chewing.

As a person learns to chew more slowly and thoroughly, he or she should observe quite frequently that this natural effect of eating properly results in a natural inclination to a normal bowel movement not long after the meal. This person should allow ample time for this bowel response or, inevitably, denial will result in constipation. **Let me stress here that the bowel urge should *never* be suppressed.**

4. Drink little fluid with your meal. Since stomach juices break down and digest food, to dilute these juices renders the digestive process more difficult. For maximum digestion, wait as long as possible after the meal before drinking anything; wait until your body craves liquid. Besides diluting your digestive juices, drinking with your meal also will cause an already overly full stomach to stretch, resulting in a distended belly. Eating too much volume, forcing the stomach to hold more than designed to hold, likewise will produce a large stomach. I have seen many people whose stomachs often retain food for as much as twenty-four hours following a meal.

5. Do not eat too much variety, too many different types of food, at a meal. The less variety at a meal, the better you will feel. In fact, a mono-diet, one food at a meal, is more palatable and digestible than a combination of foods because the body's natural instinct apparently selects one tasty food at a time. Children, if left alone, will attempt automatically to make a meal of one food—before they become perverted by a zealous parent to eat a variety of food. The stomach operates better the simpler the diet. As someone has said, "The poor stomach looked up and said, 'For goodness sakes, what's coming next?' "

6. Occasionally select a day to eat nuts only. For this purpose, include some good ones; pecans, hickory, walnuts, hazelnuts, brazil nuts, and almonds. These nuts should always be raw, unsulphured, organically or naturally grown, and should be kept refrigerated after shelling. Oils in nuts will become rancid after they have been exposed to the air for a time. You'll be surprised how a small handful of nuts can satisfy those hunger pangs, but remember to chew them thoroughly.

7. Do not cook the life out of your food. Vegetables should be cooked no longer than three minutes. A good guide to remember is "Maximum life will remain in food cooked with minimum heat and time"—the higher the heat, the more life destroyed. Most foods don't require cooking. As we begin to heat a food, we begin to destroy the life in that food. I still remember the Chinese fable I read in grade school about the origin of roasting meat:

> Apparently, one morning the swineheard, Ho-ti, went into the woods, leaving his cottage in the care of his son, Bo-bo. The boy, fond of playing with fire, let some sparks fall by accident into a bundle of straw. The fire could not be checked, and the house burned to the ground. What was worse, with the cottage perished nine little pigs.
>
> While Bo-bo was thinking what he should say to his father, an odor came to his nostrils unlike anything he had ever smelled before. He stooped down to see if there were any sign of life in the pigs and burned his fingers. To cool them, he put them into his mouth, and for the first time in his life (in the world's life, indeed), he tasted cracklings.

Digestion and Secretion

At length, the boy realized that it was the pig that smelled so savory and the pig that tasted so delicious. He fell to tearing up whole handfuls of the flesh and was cramming it down his throat when his father came and began to beat the young rogue across his shoulder. Bo-bo heeded the blows no more than if they had been flies. When he had eaten nearly all of it, he cried, "Oh, father, the pig, the pig! Do taste how nice the burnt pig is."

Father and son sat down, and never left off until they had eaten all that remained of the nine pigs. From that day, Ho-ti's cottage was always burning down. Soon, other houses in the neighborhood began to burn. Fuel and pigs became enormously costly all over the district. Finally, somebody discovered that the flesh of a pig or of any other animal might be roasted without burning down a whole house. And that, so the story goes, was how cooking began. (This story may remind us of the absurdity of cooking, especially when we do not need to do so.)

8. Eat only when you have time to relax, and are happy. Eating under stress is a major cause of indigestion. Many good books discuss how stress, hate, discontent affect the body's normal functions (see for example, *Anatomy of an Illness* by Norman Cousins, W. W. Norton & Company, Inc.) The environment for a meal should be a happy one and peaceful since excitement draws blood away from the stomach to other bodily parts, causing the stomach to perform less efficiently.

THE STOMACH

Our stomachs are remarkable organs, with walls consisting of four layers or coats:

1. An outer layer of a serous coat derived from the peritoneum;
2. A muscular coat of layers of longitudinal, transverse, and oblique muscle fibres;
3. An areolar coat consisting of loose connective tissue;
4. An inner coat composed of mucosa and containing some gastric glands. These glands secrete gastric juices—thin, watery fluid containing two to three percent hydrochloric acid and various enzymes (particularly pepsin, rennin, and gastric lipase).

This system contains all the necessary elements to conduct effective, painless, beneficial digestion in human beings (See page 19 for a Diagram of The Digestive System). Then, with nature's perfect plan to digest food for the body's use, why does food not digest properly? Why does one have stomach pains after eating? Why the chronic ailments of indigestion, and flatulence? What blocks satisfactory working of these juices on food particles? What interferes with adequate production of these digestive juices? At least five factors explain why digestion—a normally natural, beneficial, painless process—works so poorly for so many persons.

1. That most people today produce inadequate amounts of digestive juices is evident by lab tests of patients' stomach juices. Because of a minerally-poor, highly-refined diet, the muscle wall of the stomach degenerates, leaving the wall atonic and stretched. Such a stomach wall does not and will not secrete digestive juices adequately. Another indication of this lack is habitual craving for acid foods and drinks such as colas, fruit juices, and beer. In his chapter on "Vermont Folk Medicine and Beverages" (see his book *Folk Medicine*), Dr. Jarvis elaborates on the acid stomach and its need for these acids, mentioning that apple and grape vinegar seem to increase production of HCL and subsequently pepsin.

2. The oil or fat coating of fried food is difficult for digestive juices to break down.

3. In addition to attracting calcium from the blood the minute it hits the stomach, refined sugar also produces an inhibiting effect upon secretion of stomach gastric juices. Also, when eaten with proteins or starches, sugars digested in the intestine are held up in the stomach awaiting digestion of other food. The favorable, warm conditions result in fermentation, causing indigestion, sour stomach, and sour belching.

4. Because the stomach was designed by nature for a primitive diet, too much variety of food at one time places excessive demands on the stomach's overall job.

5. Too much liquid with a meal decreases the normal concentration of digestive juices, leading to inadequate digestion. Public alkaline drinking water interferes with proper secretion of digestive juices in the stomach, which leans toward the acid side. It interferes mainly with secretion of HCL, thereby interfering with secretion of pepsin—the chief active principle of gastric juice—because HCL is the forerunner of pepsin.

ABSORPTION, TRANSPORTATION, AND ASSIMILATION

From the stomach, food passes into the intestines. Here we encounter an equally fascinating organ. Instead of my paraphrasing the definition of medical, learned, and popular dictionaries, permit me to quote from *Webster's Third New International Dictionary* (Merriam-Webster, Inc., 1981):

> Intestine . . . the tubular portion of the alimentary canal that in the vertebrate lies posterior to the stomach from which it is separated by the pyloric valve and consists typically of a slender but long anterior part made up of duodenum, jejunum, and ileum which function in digestion and assimilation of nutrients and a broader shorter posterior part made up usually of cecum, colon, and rectum which serve chiefly to extract moisture from the by-products of digestion and evaporate them into feces.

This vital job of digestion and assimilation occurs after the bile from the liver and the pancreatic juices have been admitted into the small intestine, usually twenty more feet. But because of our highly-refined and mucous-

Digestion and Secretion

producing diet, a thick, tenacious, and difficult secretion forms on the wall of the small intestine, interfering with absorption of food elements. This condition, also occurring in the bowel, is an immediate problem in people with excessive mucous in their heads; those with continuous sinus drainage, recurring sore throats, voice problems, headaches, ear aches and noises, etc.

Transportation, the movement of food materials throughout the body to every cell, is a constant process. Each cell must receive food and remove poison constantly. The living cell is never dormant; the process of feeding and elimination is continuous. If man abides by all of nature's laws, this process will operate perfectly and disease-free at all times.

Assimilation, the end result, then, refers to the process of food converting into new living structure. The utlimate goal is new life in the cell, contributing to the cell's functioning, as each cell is renewed and repaired continously. In *Vermont Folk Medicine*, Dr. Jarvis explains how natural apple cider vinegar can help to change the body's chemistry, which controls the performance of the chemical laboratory within the cell.

The residue or waste portion of the food is carried from the body by the large intestine. This procedure we will discuss in chapter V, "Colon." Let me introduce, however, a few important points. Food should exit the colon in ten hours or less; normally, on a natural diet, persons have three to four good, bulky, bowel movements a day; volume content of the colon should contain ten percent residue and ninety percent bacteria; and the sign of a healthy bowel movement is a dark-brown, full stool that floats on top of the water in the bowl. To achieve and maintain this normal, healthy, rhythmic, and fully-functioning colon, one must live on a natural diet.

For a person to possess a normal appetite, it is imperative that the colon empty regularly and completely. When elimination is interfered with—as in the case of impactions—nature will tell the stomach not to be hungry, because the sewer is still full. These impactions in the colon interfere with elimination and with normal operation of all sphincters and valves, which prevent the reverse movement of anything in the colon. Thus, elimination is imperative for digestion to occur because when the brain tells the system not to eat, consequently the system likewise will not secrete the juices necessary for digestion. Normally, secretions involved in the digestive process are available only if the body enjoys a normal appetite, meaning that digestive juices are not needed except for the presence of food.

Chapter III
MEDICINE AND DISEASE: NO MYSTERY
NATURAL LAW AND WATER FLOW

Recently I visited the Cumberland Falls State Park in south-central Kentucky. As I relaxed on the patio of the lodge, I viewed the meandering Cumberland River far below, and reflected on the thundering Falls just around the bend. As I became aware of the obedience of nature, following her own law of gravitation, never trying to violate or repel that law, I reflected on the similarities of man's treatment of disease and his actions toward nature in respect to this obedience.

As a stream or river moves on unimpaired, it carries with it the silt and impurities from upstream. When dammed, however, even to prevent flooding, flooding may result either upstream or downstream. Besides disturbing the ecological balance by excessive pollution backup, the river (or lake as it soon becomes) eventually will be eliminated over a great period of time, by the same silt and materials earlier carried away by these waters.

NATURAL LAW AND THE HUMAN BODY

Frequently, we doctors fail to understand the wonders of nature as it constantly works to right society's wrongs. Men and women attempt to blame their failure on nature.

You cannot break God's natural laws concerning bodily health and not receive adverse reactions, any more than you can expect to drive your car down the road at high speed, hit a large object head-on, and not expect to be harmed physically. Any action will create a reaction, and when that action changes or interferes with a natural law, then that reaction will almost always be adverse. The body is constantly on the offense, demonstrating its inborn facility to correct violations of natural law.

In administering to the sick, we are taught commonly that illness is a violent attack on the human body from without. What we actually witness is the body's power to rid itself of, or correct, a wrong or some violation of natural law.

Doctors today play at treating disease. In the old game of "Mud Pies" I used to play as a child, we pretended that the mud pies we patted out were real. We would go to great lengths to mix them, form them, bake them, set them on the table, and sit down to eat them. All done in pretense, of course. Today's doctors are playing "Mud Pie" because they treat the patient's symptoms instead of treating causes of disease. Nature's laws, in action, appear meaningless. We doctors are trained to suppress scientific performance of the body trying to heal itself—which it always will do if it possesses the proper fuel or elements it should receive through food, water, and air, and if all the avenues of waste escape work properly so that the body can utilize these totally.

The body is the most scientifically created machine in the universe as we know it. The human body was structured by natural law, operates by natural law, and will operate perfectly if we follow that natural law.

During the early 1930's, I studied under Dr. Pearson at Kirksville College of Osteopathic Medicine: He taught that *"disease is the process of getting well!"* Little did I understand, then, how much truth he stated.

SYMPTOM AND CAUSE

So much variation exists in definitions of disease or disease states that it confuses doctors and laymen alike. Today, we classify disease by naming it according to symptoms or, often, by naming it after the person who classified it. In most cases, a disease manifestation is named according to certain signs a person sees under specific conditions when, actually, the body is exerting effort to return to its normal state.

This named set of symptoms or manifestations should only *qualify* the conditions as to the *cause*. The point I hope to stress and clarify here is that most conditions, called diseases, are not the disease at all, but rather are visible or obvious objective recovery efforts of the body. *The disease should be known by what has already occurred before the symptoms ever developed.* Therefore, we should direct our treatment to the primary cause and not to the symptom.

THE DIAGNOSIS: FROM SYMPTOM TO CAUSE

It follows naturally that the patient and the doctor should think backward from symptoms to cause to determine treatment, for the symptom (often called the disease) invariably will disappear when the cause is corrected. This process will become clear as we discuss specific diseases.

It is virtually impossible to find a book large enough to contain every disease known by the symptom-complex name. For instance, we are told that more than 2,000 varieties of one type of virus exist which can produce numerous specifically named influenzas. How can the human mind possibly determine which brand of flu a person has?

This idea, "the error in diagnosis," is by no means original with me. Others have proposed it usually along the same line of thought: Disease naming should derive from descriptions and chemical and physical derangements of the body, (by etiology, the cause).

CONDITIONS WHICH PRODUCE ALL SYMPTOMS

We must realize that *all* symptom complexes result from the *same* following conditions:

Medicine and Disease: No Mystery

1. Presence of waste matter or toxins in the body;
2. Absence of pure, fresh, poison-free substance in the body. That is, elements of nature, living foods, are necessary to feed the body for it to perform as nature designed; and
3. The inevitable need to correct all chemical and structural abnormalities in the body.

When these three condtions are not adhered to, we violate natural law.

Since we are told that science is truth, we think unscientifically if we otherwise view diagnosis of disease. It would be easier for a scientist to prove that "germs" *do not* cause disease than it would be to attempt to prove that they *do* cause disease.

Frequently, doctors are so puzzled—trying to fit a symptom complex to a disease name—that they become frustrated. This frustration doctors transmit to patients, who already may feel ill and despondent, when told "We can find nothing wrong with you."

I have seen many cases of gastro-intestinal complaints, examined through usual diagnostic procedures, end up with negative reports. Later, however, following a more thorough, intensive internal examination, these same cases invariably showed abnormalities in their gastro-intestinal chemistry flora and/or showed severe structural abnormalities of internal organs and structures.

Some people believe they are "a victim of disease," as if disease purposely chose that particular person. Others brag that they were attacked by a germ, a virus, or some other mystical agent.

If we actually "catch something that's going around" (as we often say), then we should constantly all be "catching something that's going around" all the time. Logically, therefore, all people would have all diseases, all the time.

There are seasons when it does seem that we all are "catching something"—particularly, for example, in the flu season. But you will not suffer from flu if your body does not *need the flu*. It is impossible to "catch" anything unless your body is a fertile field for scavengers, such as germs or viruses, needed to remove bodily waste.

The symptom of the runny nose, for example, implies that the body is overloaded with waste and is attempting to wash out the waste with its own scavenger system. The amount of overload is proportionate to the degree of swelling, secretions, and other symptoms. Logical treatment, then, would be to assist the eliminative system as it attempts to unload.

Our usual procedure, however, is to suppress this evidence by taking a pain killer and/or to take a drug to kill the invader which caused the disease, which also can destroy the body's immune power to function and to repair. Moreover, such drugs will add more strain to the body as it attempts to eliminate them since these drugs are not natural elements the body is equipped to utilize.

Vaccines constitute other forms of matter foreign to the body which also must be eliminated. I was taught and trained that the smallpox vaccine was effective, safe, necessary. According, however, to an *AMA Journal* article (reprint, *Prevention Magazine*), smallpox vaccination is not necessary. The book, *Bacteria, Incorporated* by Cash Asher, exposes how the health department in San Antonio, Texas, some years ago, discovered that smallpox was found only where bedbugs existed, and where there were no bedbugs, there also was no smallpox.

During the early 1980's, along with other physicians, I was asked to participate in a massive innoculation, supposedly to prevent a certain strain of flu epidemic. Naturally, I refused because nature told me many times during my forty-six years of experience, that nature only requires an illness when the body needs it. Knowing and believing that nature's laws are inviolable, I had no right participating in artificially producing an unnatural state of so-called immunity. Even if I had believed that the body was attacked by flu, I thought it difficult for any physician to determine which flu strain to protect against. During the same period as the expected epidemic (which to this day has not occurred), a scientific article appearing in our local newspaper stated that one type of flu caused by a virus appeared in more than 2,000 varieties, or strains. It is inconceivable to me that a finite mind could determine which of 2,000 varieties of flu could attack a person before this person knew he or she was even going to become ill.

The mass innoculation, however, did occur, funded by our federal government, which has since faced over one billion dollars worth of law suits filed against it because of the sequence of events following these shots, particularly from the substantial incidence of paralysis. During this time, I was called to attend one of the victims, a young mother paralyzed from the neck down after receiving her flu shot.

This case also reminds me of a friend's daughter who developed multiple sclerosis. This girl had been revaccinated during her early years more than fifteen times, because the law required an innoculation before a person could enter school regardless of how many tries needed before the vaccination succeeded. Since that time, I have read many similar stories, some in medical literature, suggesting that the smallpox vaccination seems to be related to the incidence of multiple sclerosis.

Why has the public become so gullible, so ready to accept the professional's word? If the wrong people were in power, a mass innoculation could wipe out an entire society. It is fear of disease, dread of heart trouble, horror of cancer, etc. that compels us to grasp any thread of hope we can. In Hebrews 2, Paul wrote that God placed all things in subjection—power and control—to and under human beings. Disease was not meant as a force to overcome people, but as a force for people which people must understand. We can free ourselves from fear of disease if we understand disease.

Sickness is the body's response or reaction to environmental and self-imposed violations of natural laws. If the body did not respond, it would,

Medicine and Disease: No Mystery

most certainly, become more vulnerable to destruction. When the body reacts, it evidences an offense to correct those errors and violations.

It is an historical, medical fact that Jewish people, during the Dark Ages in Europe, did not contract nor succumb to epidemics then raging throughout Europe. Some historians have reasoned that the Jews remained immune because they adhered to God's biological laws relative to foods they ate. It is also a known fact that today tribes of people in various parts of the world do not suffer from epidemics (for detailed studies, see *A Study of the Healthy Hunza of Asia*, by Dr. Allen Banik; *Bacteria, Inc.*, by Cash Asher; *Diet Prevents Polio*, by Dr. Benjamin Sandler).

Finally, it is established fact, admitted by these people and doctors alike, that Seventh Day Adventists in America, who live by these biological laws, enjoy the highest state of health of any Christian group in America. You know of persons enjoying a noticeable degree of better health than the general population. If the culprit is "germs," then why aren't we all sick all the time? Just what role do "germs" play in the picture of health?

Germs or viruses have the same position as insects in plant life. Germs were created for human beings, not against human beings, as stated in the first chapter of Genesis. Germs belong to the plant kingdom, given to us, for our good; therefore, we should not consider them "a cause of disease" but as scavenger agents to remove from the body what is foreign to the body habitat. They function in the balance of nature, the "Circle of Health." (For an investigation of this concept, see *One Hundred Million Guinea Pigs* by Paul DeKruf.)

Your body machine, literally laboratory, always knows what is going on, and constantly tries to adjust to many different conditions. It is, therefore, contrary to nature and to science for human beings to treat and to attempt to obliterate symptoms instead of trying to correct causes of symptoms. You cannot correct a situation by refusing to admit the situation exists.

To mask or prevent a symptom is not truly *medicine* if, in fact, medicine actually means the science and art of dealing with the prevention, cure, or alleviation of disease—that part of the science and art of restoring and preserving health customarily the physician's province.

In *Sugar Blues*, William Dufty explains the "mystery" of medicine. In his chapter on "How We Got Here from There," Dufty explains how early priests used Latin names to make a disease sound mysterious, how doctors wrote prescriptions in Latin for their patients so they would not know what they were taking, and how doctors enforced the idea of medicine's mystery. There is no mystery to it. Health follows exact natural law. When we attempt, however, to improve on God, on his law—to do it our way—we sin and must suffer the consequences (because we sin, when we are not anchored in God's law, in union with his laws). If mystery exists, it concerns our tendency to sin, not our body's tendency to survive well.

Recently, I heard a doctor tell a group of students that there has never been one drug that ever cured any one disease: "Even drug companies admit it. Do you know the actual action of an aspirin? Now aspirin is common, you all use it. Do you know how it works?" Not one hand went up. Nobody knew how an aspirin works. He continued, "There, you see, you don't know how any drug works. You don't even know what it does to the body. If you did, you wouldn't use it. Even the drug companies will admit that they only know what a drug does by its action through the symptom of the patient."

We are a drug-oriented society; a large portion of advertising aims at drug and medicine-related products. A pain hits; we reach for a drug. Not long ago I heard a popular late-night TV comedian kidding about doctors. I chuckled when he commented: "They're called 'wonder drugs' because the doctor rubs his chin, frowns, and says, 'I wonder which one I should use this time.'"

It is natural law for the body to heal itself. It will always attempt to heal, and it will always try to return to normal, regardless of what you do. In this healing effort, it will follow exactly the laws of science. Only when we interfere with these laws do we get into trouble.

PAIN AS SIGNAL

Human bodies operate analogically, as automobiles do. Automobiles operate according to scientific law. If they didn't, you would never arrive at your destination. You care for your vehicle by maintaining it, or soon you will have no vehicle. You repair your vehicle, applying the laws or mechanic's instructions for that vehicle. You don't repair a car with bicycle repair instructions. You discover your car needs repairs by its symptoms, whether a squeak, groan, explosion, foul odor, or inability to start.

As with a car and its symptoms, body pain indicates the body needs repair. As a sign, it points to something wrong. Pain results from obstruction preventing movement. Nearly always, I have found that the cause of pain can be located and corrected. Pain indicates the body's attempts to overcome some problem. Another cause of pain could be pressure on a nerve, or the nerve could be in a bad chemical environment, irritating it and causing pain. Pain is felt through the sensory nerve, the one detecting what is wrong. It is an indicator like your automobile gas gauge. Or more realistically, we can compare a pain signal to the red danger light on your automobile's front drive panel when this light indicates the car is overheated and could explode any time. The motor nerves transmit electrical impulses that make some body part work, as in a contraction. The sensory nerves register impressions or images of a part in trouble. Pain indicates trouble. Thus, it is extremely unscientific to deaden pain but not to find the cause of that pain.

FEVER AS SIGNAL

Fever also illustrates the healing process and is produced by body needs. Fever can result from the presence of an overloaded intestine. This observation can be proven easily through repeated enemas until the bowel unloads. We use biological and physiological aids such as vinegar, lemon juice, sorghum, acidophilus cultures, and sea salt added to water. Normally, enema water

Medicine and Disease: No Mystery

should approximate normal body temperature, but if a person happens to be chilling at the time, then it would be well to use warmer water; likewise, if the patient is too hot, then cooler water could be used. We use these proportions for our patients:
 1 tablespoon vinegar to 1 pint water
 pure sorghum or honey - 2 tablespoons to 1 pint water
 liquid acidophilus - 2 ounces undiluted
 sea salt - 1 tablespoon to 1 pint water.

Fever should never be dangerous and always benefits: We should utilize it to strengthen the body. An American university worked with volunteer prisoners in an artificial fever test, keeping these men's temperatures at 110 degrees for days without apparent harm. Convulsions, claimed to result from excessive fever, are caused by body toxins—primarily in the large intestine. Fever was considered beneficial for more than 2,000 years, until aspirin was discovered. Many cultures used sweat houses or encouraged high fever for all types of ailments which fever accompanied, including syphilis and tuberculosis.

How Fever Works Beneficially

When the body becomes overloaded with toxins and fever is necessary to aid in their elimination, the hypothalamus, which regulates the body's temperature, raises the body's thermostat. The body, now cooler than the thermostat or hypothalamus indicates that it should be, raises its body temperature to compensate. Nerve messages originating in the hypothalamus trigger rapid muscle contractions, or shivering, which causes heat production. When the fever center is alerted to act, the following occurs:

1. Heart rate increases to promote more rapid removal of foreign bodies by the blood;
2. Increasing body heat also causes blood vessels to dilate, radiating more warmth everywhere in the body, and by creating more vascular space, provides more room for blood to act on toxins.

This increased volume of blood space operates much the same as flood waters going in every direction to pick up more debris, cleansing the land by 'washing' from the moving water.

In simpler words, fever burns body waste faster. Therefore, we can say truthfully that fever always helps (for good) and never harms. The body will shut off automatically the fever signal when *increased* temperature and circulation no longer are needed.

Illness, disease, sickness, affliction—call it whatever you like—our society seems built on its cause, its proliferation, and its cure. Government subsidizes us when we are sick; we invest in insurance to guarantee us the best medical care; movies and books are based on incurable illnesses; and the topic of many conversations is a hospital visit or operation. This nation's state of health (or rather "ill-health") seems to be our new "God." I need not tell you about medicine's high cost today, or about the highly advanced technology "necessary" for treatment of disease. Medical costs are so high today that the average citizen cannot even afford health insurance premiums. Daily we are informed of cancer research, DNA research, heart research, advances in artificial organs and joints, etc. How often do we hear about funding research for preventive medicine or for diseases perhaps caused by deficiency? What would happen to all the research centers if it were proven by a government- or private-funded research project that all diseases were related definitely to toxins and deficiencies and that pure food, water, and air could maintain a totally healthy population?

We cannot see the forest for the trees. Are we so sophisticated that we cannot recognize the simple? Or does simple human nature cause us to place the blame elsewhere—on the germ, or on being 'hit' or 'attacked' by a stroke, a coronary, or other ailment? You are neither hit nor attacked; rather *you* are the primary cause of your own problem. You are responsible for your ailment. A body *problem* is not *only* in the head or elbow, or the stomach, or big toe but also frequently is connected or related to some other part or parts of the entire body.

We do know many answers to questions about preventing bad health. I was in a store owned by parents of a young child recently dead from a blood disease. After the child's death, these parents were willing to give away everything they owned to advance research to find the cause of their child's illness. Their well-intentioned idea was to prevent the same thing from happening to other children. I have also a close friend whose wife suffered from a degenerative, central nervous system disease. I often hear him boast that he is most interested in funding research into the cause of his wife's problem, at any cost. I observe these people and others like them, eating devitalized foods known to cause the same diseases in test animals they wish to cure. These same people find it difficult to recognize the simple fact that diet and disease are related.

We were not meant to be so afflicted, nor is it necessary that we die from horrible disease. Reconstructive surgery, originating from the war years and now much advanced, is often unnecessary. The body can and does recover and regenerate. We do not have to live in fear of today's dreaded diseases.

Responsibility lies with us all. If I know the cause or causes of a person's problem and have not done all in my power to prevent or help to eliminate that problem, I am responsible. As the old proverb goes, "If I know of an evil and do nothing in my power to overcome that evil, then I am an accomplice to that evil."

You must examine your responsibility to yourself, as I must recognize my responsibility to you. Your responsibility is to seek, to study, to discover, and to understand what you have done to violate nature's laws that results in your bodily problems. Then when you have learned and can accept these ideas, it is your God-given duty to correct all you can for yourself. If I am acquainted with you or can reach you with information and knowledge, it is

Medicine and Disease: No Mystery

my duty to inform you regarding causes of your problems and what you can do about them.

Though a cliché, it rings true (as clichés often do): A chain is only as strong as its weakest link. In today's society, we cannot afford weak links because they soon may result in a broken chain in which we all become victims.

Chapter IV

DETOXIFICATION

One of the most potent, yet simple, ways to de-toxify is to fast. I recommend that everyone acquire one or more books on fasting, and fast at least one day a week. A good assortment of books relating to fasting usually can be found at any natural food store, some large book stores, or libraries.

Some reasons and advantages of fasting include the following:

1. Fasting will cause your food to taste better;
2. Fasting will prevent your stomach from becoming enlarged—out of proportion. Nearly all stomachs are too big, and hold too much food. One reason for an enlarged stomach may—indeed, likely—will result from many years on a refined diet. An enlarged stomach, however, will draw up and become smaller when you fast regularly and eat less; and
3. Fasting also allows your blood time to cleanse your body better, providing it more time to unload and to rejuvenate.

Lower animals intuitively fast, if they have overeaten or eaten something wrong. But the human being has lost his instinct to recognize what is actual food, to know when to eat and when not to. Eating refined foods has resulted in significant blurring of the human being's instinct to recognize nutritional, wholesome food.

Most important, persons should drink considerable quantities of fluids while fasting; the water should be pure spring water or distilled water. It is well to caution that distilling water makes it more alkaline. Be conscious of and obey your body's craving or demand for fluid. It will guide you on the quantity it requires. These fluids aid the intestinal tract to cleanse and help to dilute toxins in the blood. By increasing your blood flow with pure water, you help it to transport these poisons out of your system faster.

Another excellent means of eliminating poisions or detoxifying (a method used frequently at our clinic) is raw rhubarb juice. Rhubarb has been known for a long time to help the liver to work better. Many years ago, some popular laxative pills were made with rhubarb (or rhubarb root). The juice of the rhubarb plant is a cholagogue, which means it stimulates production of bile by liver cells. Rhubarb juice works in the same manner on the pancreas.

Bile is one of the digestive juices dumped into the small intestine immediately after food leaves the stomach; mainly in this intestine it works on all food substances. Bile also is the natural laxative that keeps the food from becoming dormant or stagnant as it moves through the body—the means of transportation, so to speak.

The rhubarb treatment procedure we use is as follows:

We take a fresh, large diameter-sized, piece of rhubarb—3 or 4 inches long—and blend it with enough apple juice to make an 8-ounce liquid drink. If too sour, and the patient desires it sweeter, we add a small teaspoon or more of pure honey. Then the patient drinks all 8 ounces at once. The rhubarb causes the bile to secrete and fill the gall bladder, which automatically empties as required by the food stream passing through the small intestine. One to two hours later, the patient drinks all-at-once 4 ounces of olive oil blended with 4 ounces of apple juice. As the oil leaves the stomach, it passes over the opening of the common bile duct, where it empties into the small intestine, triggering the valve to open and the gall bladder to contract. This triggering action is caused by the oil fat. Then, I advise my patients to continue this oil-rhubarb treatment, once a week for a month, and I advise them to ingest a natural herbal laxative every other day until they are well-cleaned out. When the stool becomes brown and less light in color, the patient knows that the gall bladder is emptying after it is filled by the liver juice.

After the first month of the rhubarb-oil treatment, the patient rests the second month, using no treatment. Then the third month, the patient again undergoes the same procedure as in the first month. If the reader desires to practice this method of detoxification, I advise that the person consult with a doctor regarding frequency of treatment.

The next step in detoxifying—following rhubarb-oil and herbal laxative—is to attract waste within the bowel and neutralize it with an aid which adsorbs and absorbs. Two of the best products to achieve this goal are bentonite and montmorillonite—both a volcanic ash. The trade names of these are "Veico" distributed by Veico Products, Inc. and "Natural Relief" distributed by Whole Natural Earth Products. These products (and possibly other brands of the same content) a person can find in most natural food stores. I advise my patients to take a dose, as directed on the bottle, three times a day for one month.

This treatment helps to clean more than would be cleaned otherwise. An explanation on the "Sonne's #7" container, another brand bentonite, describes the product as an adsorbent aid in detoxification and intestinal purification via the alimentary canal.

Detoxification, or cleansing, is important to health maintenance especially when various threats to good health exist within the body—as the next chapters indicate.

Chapter V

COLON

Most standard and technical dictionaries define the colon as extending from the cecum to the rectum. The human colon divides into 1) the ascending colon (rising on the abdomen's right side), 2) transverse colon (crossing from the left to right side), 3) the descending colon (descending on the left side), and 4) the sigmoid colon (a labyrinthine portion which becomes continuous with the rectum). Figure 1 displays the human digestive system and the internal relationships of one part to another. You may wish to view this system as preparation for what follows (See Figure 1).

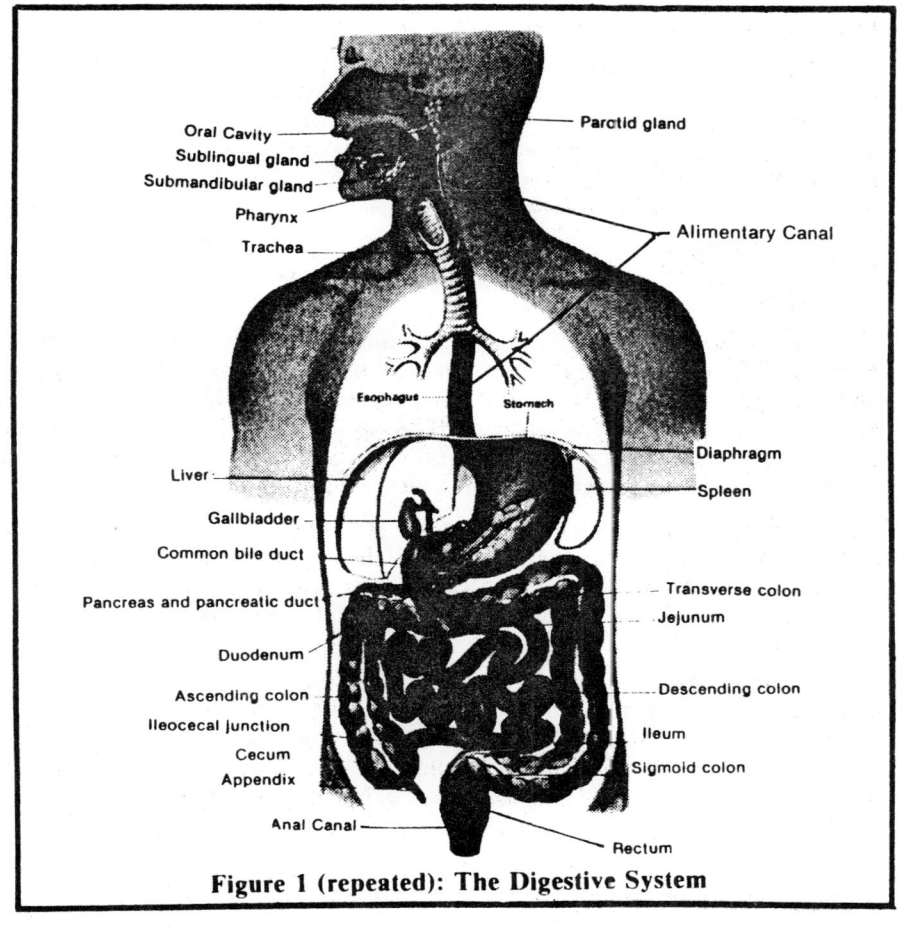

Figure 1 (repeated): The Digestive System

The dominant symptom in more than ninety percent of all patients first visiting my clinic indicates the colon as the origin. Described as the window to the body, the colon is the most informative part of the body. All my patients undergo colon examination, usually a colonic, and as a result, further colon treatment (most patients will require such). Some of my more jocular patients delight in referring to me as "Captain Colonic." (One patient even wrote a poem on that caption!)

Today, people are bowel conscious because of the common disturbance of constipation. The term "constipation" bears a broader meaning than merely daily bowel elimination. Actually, anything short of complete evacuation is constipation, a condition most common today.

In observing elimination by animals living on nature's foods (raw foods which man likewise was designed to eat), we learn that these animals frequently eliminate. Man, however, inclines to think he is a different organism, needing to eliminate only after considerable time.

Some years ago, *Nervous Indigestion*, a popular medical text book appeared and taught that human daily elimination is not necessary. This book referred to a physical fitness teacher, a lady who had one massive evacuation a week. As a long-time student of nature, I say that this routine is insufficient and that weekly elimination results from the bowel's degenerative condition, characteristic of our society.

JOBS OF THE COLON

Often overlooked but important, the colon's normal chemistry produces enzymes. These enzymes, produced in the colon, are absorbed by the lymph and then absorbed into the blood which transports them to stimulate and activate various body cells and glands. Also, some enzymes formed in the colon, produced by the flora (bacteria), are used there. Here they assist in production of stool material for the colon's physiology or mobility.

The colon, designed to absorb certain food elements, can absorb toxic materials or poisons, one good reason the colon should empty often, probably six, eight, or ten hours after eating. An example of this absorption is the experiment where a clove of garlic inserted into the rectum affects taste in the mouth within sixteen seconds.

The rectum, the final portion of the colon, should never contain any fecal matter except during a bowel movement. If a person suppresses bowel urges continually, fecal matter will move into the rectum until the person has lost the urge, resulting in habitual constipation. This problem becomes intensified, then, because habit allows absorption from the rectum.

The colon prepares the food residue by mixing it in segments—one small portion to the next—and by massive mixing, moving it forward and backward, a churning motion by the individual saculations or parts, while combining it with the enzymes and bacteria in the colon, and then forming it into the stool. This action results from the peristaltic movements. These movements are peculiar wormlike wave motions of the intestines and other similar structure, produced by successive contractions of muscular fibers of their walls, forcing the contents forward. The human peristalsis involves a centrifugal movement in each segment, a massive movement of one part of the colon to the next, and then a reverse movement. As a person loses the tone of the colon from degeneration, it affects the peristalsis by reducing the muscle and nerve control of the muscle that creates the peristalsis.

Involved in the colon's mechanical operation is a normal acid colon chemistry. Necessary factors such as bulky materials and presence of numerous bacteria stimulate colon movement. That is, they *all* enter into the contraction and the churning of the colon wall.

THE RECTUM AND ELIMINATION

I have observed that persons eating raw, living foods do eliminate often, as animals do. Therefore, I would suggest that in most people it is natural and necessary to have at least three movements daily.

Today, we commonly find persons retaining in their colon food residue or filler they have eaten the previous week—a deplorable situation. From my years of practice, however, it has become evident to me that a diet of live whole food will result in the residue remaining in the bowel no more than six, eight, or ten hours at the most. By the end of that period, the food should be well-utilized and composted by your sewer department, the colon, leaving the colon ready to begin the circle of health again. This circle of health also includes the natural law that requires man to replenish the earth with body residue from both bowel and bladder.

COLON DIAGNOSES

Most people recognize the problem of constipation. In addition, doctors can observe certain, significant conditions:

1. A turgescent wall, one with a regenerative, inflamed, or engorged appearance, which means the bowel is attempting to regenerate;
2. Tumors, such as polyps and cancerous growths: These cancerous growths, within the colon (in the lumen or colon space) are distinguished by their proclivity to bleeding;
3. Varicose veins (in the colon wall) and hemorrhoids which become sources of bleeding;
4. Evidence of ulcers and craters where ulcers have been and healed; and
5. The most common occurrence, however, is the scale and other impacted material adhering to the colon's inner wall, often for a lengthy time.

Other conditions not visible to the doctor's eye, but visible on x-ray include ptosis, wall contour change, and colon elongation from mineral lack.

PTOSIS

Ptosis represents a fallen condition of the abdominal organ. If we graded the degree of ptosis by numbers 1-4, evidently most cases of ptosis from the teen-age years on fall in category 3. This number means that the bowels have fallen ¾ as far as possible in the abdominal cavity. Some persons believe a dropped colon has little to do with their condition. On the contrary, it is important—as evidenced by the relieved and uplifted feelings of patients when their organs are supported by a ptosis appliance. The most common ptosis support to hold the bowel while allowing body ligaments to pull it up is a Hastings-type ptosis support. Figures 2 and 3 illustrate frontal and back views of ptosis support. This support is worn on the lower part of the abdomen to lift up the viscera (abdominal organs).

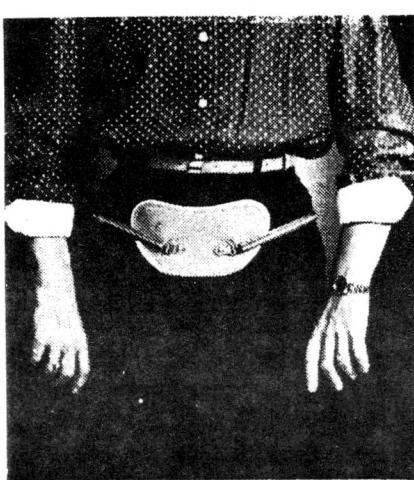

Figure 2: The Ptosis support (Front view)

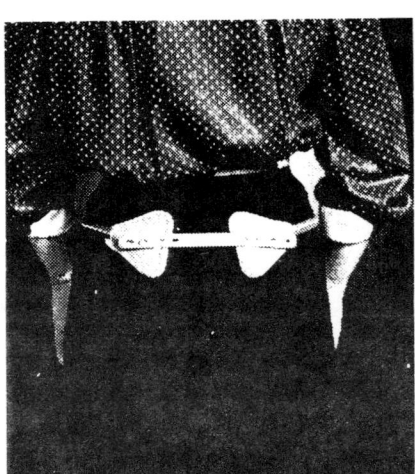

Figure 3: The Ptosis support (Back view)

WALL CONTOUR CHANGE

Change in the colon's contour wall is observable by x-ray. This commonly diagnosed condition is termed spastic colon or diverticulosis. It consists of a degenerative change of the total wall—the muscle and all—which becomes full of fibrous tissue. Fibrous tissue is similar to threadlike material, harder than normal tissue and feels ropey. This fibrous tissue makes the bowel tight. Though the body never does anything contrary to nature, nevertheless, fibrous tissue will shorten man's time on earth.

A spastic colon is not necessarily spastic; rather it is a permanent narrowing from fibrous tissue which nature deposits to reinforce the gut wall which has degenerated, replacing the normal protein structure.

Physicians can treat this condition (and, consequently, patients can learn about elimination) by tilting the body upside down, vertically, so that the abdominal content can be manipulated—loosening upward toward the diaphragm. (One excellent method of tilting is with a backswing. See Figure 4.)

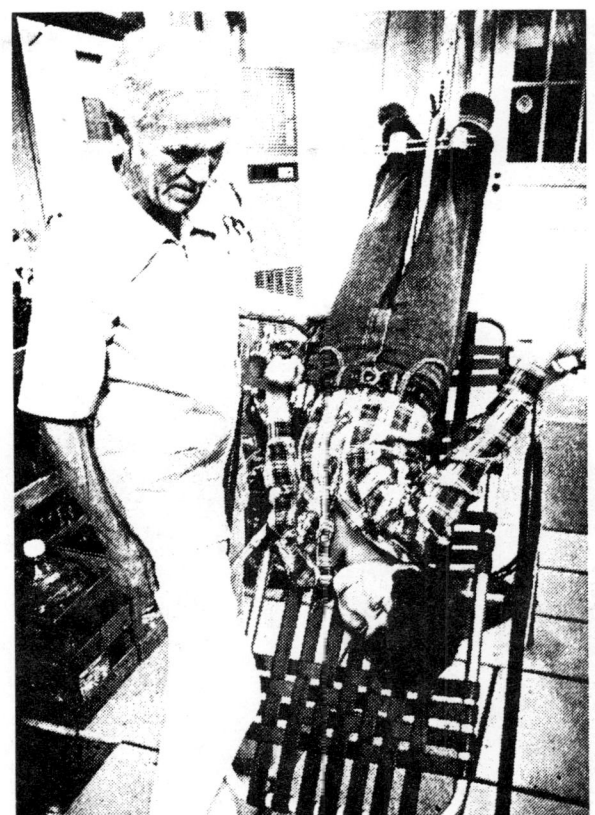

Figure 4: Dr. Robertson instructs a young asthma patient, Brandy Wilhite, on the backswing.

COLON ELONGATION FROM MINERAL LACK

Colon elongation from lack of minerals allows degeneration to develop (See pages 44-45, Figures 5 & 6, diagram of normal and abnormal colons), producing extra loops and obstructions in the looping and causing a partial volvulus or volvulus (total obstruction). Ordinarily, colon regeneration and shortening proceeds slowly. Occasionally, however, I am surprised at the speed with which a colon will regenerate and shorten on proper diet. I recall, for example, the case of the doctor who asked me to x-ray his colon again after one month's treatment. We were both shocked and amazed at the amount of regeneration.

If a person has eaten demineralized food long enough, another consequence appears: loss of normal colon structure or texture. This loss causes the colon to stretch, much like a small balloon. You may recall from your own childhood how a balloon stretches and eventually loses its tone if continuously inflated.

As the colon elongates, it must go someplace, hence the looping and falling condition.

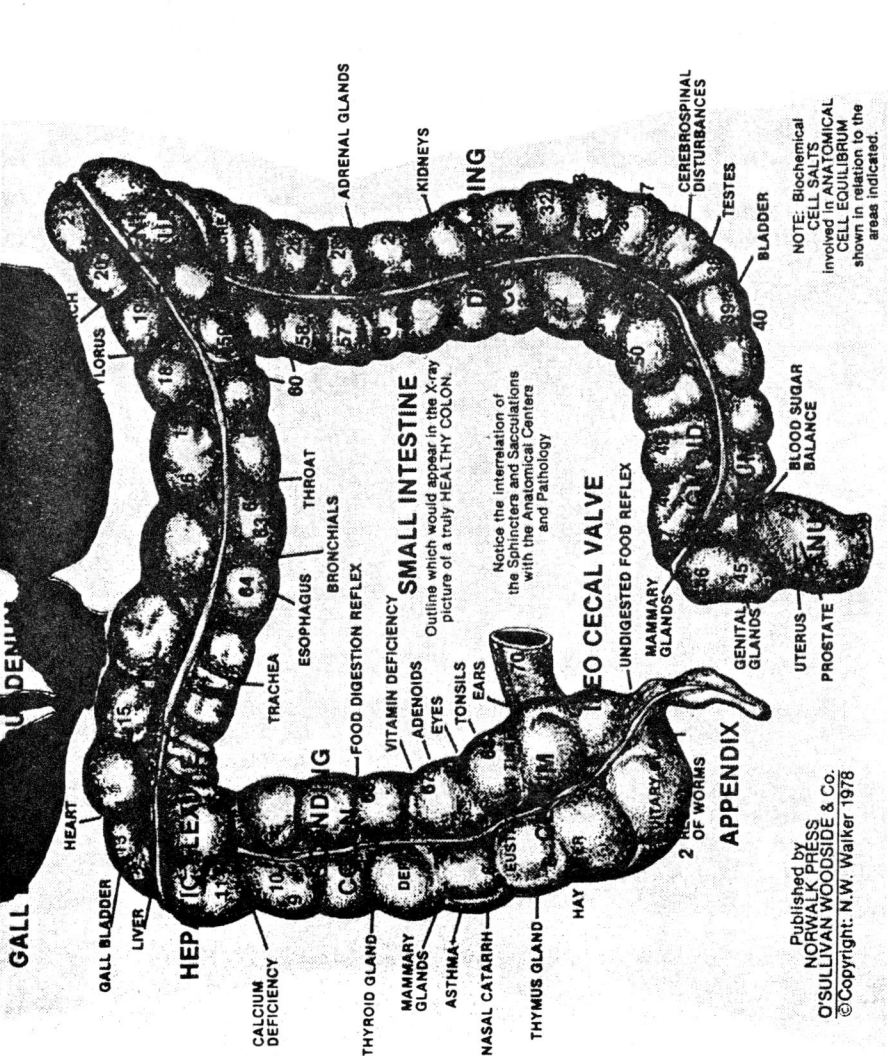

Figure 5: Healthy Colon

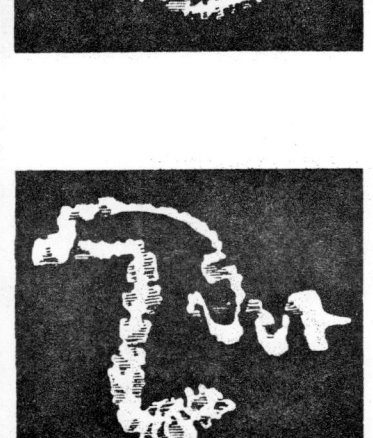

Figure 6: Sick Colons

The above six pictures of prolapsed, distorted, twisted, sickly looking colons are exact reproductions of X-ray negatives of the colons of apparently healthy, civilized people whose illusions about their physical condition were exploded when they saw this conclusive evidence. This chart has been prepared by Dr. N. W. Walker for the guidance, benefit and use by colon irrigation and lavage establishment operators, and for the education of the layman.

Civilized life means an artificial life; civilized people, living in a civilized manner and eating civilized foods, cannot, in the very nature of things, have a truly HEALTHY COLON. Health and sickness both have their roots in the COLON.

At the same time the colon wall deteriorates, supporting ligaments and tissue holding the colon in place also deteriorate, allowing the structure to fall with the aid of gravity.

EXTERNAL MANUAL TREATMENT

To help restore healthy conditions, physicians can employ several methods.

Slant Board or Degravitizer

To counter gravity's effect, one can use a slant board, or better still, a total degravitizer. As mentioned earlier, one such degravitizer is the backswing, positioning the body upside down and perpendicular to the floor:

To assist this restoration to the original position, the fixed position of the fallen organ needs to be loosened with the hands lifting upward, with the use of a vibrator, or other means. In some cases, however, because of previous surgery and developing post-surgical adhesions, a person may need to resort again to surgery to cut these adhesions. Adhesions and fibrous tissue (previously discussed) are pathologically similar.

In this manual treatment of the fallen organs, one may use finger tips or knuckles, or if a second party does it, the heel of the hand. I would suggest a doctor do the greater part of this restoration and ask him to instruct on how to follow through.

Diet

The diet must be corrected to supply elements necessary for regeneration. For full discussion, please refer to the chapter on diet, where I recommend fresh, raw, poison-free foods, and pure water and air.

For centuries, ever since man began to cook, people intuitively have degravitized the body to correct these same conditions. They also intuitively knew to cleanse the colon at times, or to purge the intestinal tract by means of herbs and fasting. You may recall that cleansing and fasting are frequently mentioned throughout the Bible.

Colon Cleansing

Today, there are many methods of colon cleansing. In this book's chapter on Detoxification, you will find Fasting and Detoxifiers discussed. From natural food stores one may purchase aids such as herbal laxatives, made from natural herbs, and bulky materials such as psyllium and flax seed. To enhance further colon normalization, acidophilus may be taken orally or used as a rectal implant to restore normal flora.

Readers may find it helpful to learn about other methods our clinic utilizes to cleanse colons. Most colons I examine look like the inside of an old garbage can never cleaned out. To clean this mess, we use enemas and colonics. As you and I both know, it is not natural to take an enema. But because man has degenerated so much, an enema aids immensely. The muscle wall may be so deficient, so degenerated, that it doesn't have the power to empty the colon on time: Thus, water from the enema or colonic helps expedite this emptying process.

Colon

The colonic is more effective because its action is like a machine gun, instead of a one-shot BB gun (as in the enema procedure). The enema, however, does have distinct advantages. To loosen colon scale and old deposits, we use several types.

Aloe Vera Enema. The aloe vera enema is made by injecting two to four ozs. of liquid aloe vera into the rectum and leaving it. The body will absorb some of it, and the remaining amount will loosen the colon scale or dead wall.

Honey Enema. The honey enema (four tablespoons of honey to one pint of water) will accomplish the same thing. Aloe is used because of its food value to the colon and because of its detoxifying effect. Honey is used because it helps feed the flora and corrects the PH toward the acid side.

Vinegar Enema. We also use a vinegar enema (one tablespoon of vinegar to one pint of water; lemon juice may substitute if vinegar is not available, but the vinegar is preferable). This enema will help to loosen scales as well as to feed and to promote better bacterial growth. The vinegar helps create and sustain the colon's normal chemistry.

Vegetable Oil Enema. A good lubricant to loosen decayed deposits around the colon wall is vegetable oil. Vegetable oils mix well with the secretion around the colon wall. We do *not* use mineral oil: it tends to coat the colon wall. Usually, one pint of vegetable oil is enough for this oil enema, with ten drops of vinegar added as desired. This oil enema should be held for two hours. While the oil remains in the colon, it helps to employ hands and fingers or fists to work around the course of the colon. This area includes the abdomen at the waist and below. Work upwards, on the right side from the bottom of the pelvis, up toward the ribs on the right, across toward the left side, and then proceed down the left side. Upon completing this sequence, reverse the process.

OTHER TREATMENTS

A good treatment helpful in restoring colon mobility and muscle tone in the bowel wall is to alternate hot and cold packs on the abdomen. To do this procedure, rub vinegar into the abdomen wall through the skin, and then place a hot steaming turkish towel on the abdomen, keeping it hot for twenty minutes. To maintain the heat, you can either cover the towel or reapply it as it cools; you can place a heat lamp over the towel, carefully placing it not so close that it will burn; or you could place a hot water bottle over the towel to keep it warm. After twenty minutes, replace the heat pack with an ice pack and leave it on from three to five minutes. Then reapply the heat pack for twenty minutes and likewise again the ice pack, repeating this sequence at least two or more times. This application of hot and cold stimulates blood supply to the bowel and all abdominal organs. An important organ is the mesentery, which carries the blood to and from the bowel and contains the nerve supply and lymph system.

THE COLON AND BACK PAIN

After some of these treatments, our patients notice they no longer suffer the back and leg pains they had for years. Let me explain.

Most everyone, now and then, suffers the lower back pain, usually labelled a back problem. To the contrary, if the sufferer reflects, he or she will discover a close correlation between back pain and a bowel problem. In my practice, I have observed a generally constant association between the two. If then, these two conditions are associated, logically we should look to the body's disposal system, primarily the gut, for the answer. The proper approach would be to have some trained person (a qualified doctor or a mother at home) analyze the bowel. Basically, it would be wise to see that the lower bowel is emptying properly. If then, when the bowel is emptied, one finds any relief to the back pain, reasonably, we may consider the bowel as the source of the problem.

It is fact that many or most degenerative bone problems produce little or no pain in the back except in the presence of toxins carried within the colon.

Thus, you fight nature when you take a drug to cover or mask back pain. The pain is the body's indication that a problem may exist in the gut and that the body is striving to correct the problem. This process is called viscero-somatic-reflex, meaning the reference from the internal organ to the surface.

THE COLON AND BACTERIA

A serious situation today—not realized by most people—is the meager residue from bowels of civilized people. When compared to bowel residue in native tribes in many parts of the world, the total bulk in their elimination is many times greater than ours. Where does this greater bulk originate?

Estimates indicate about ninety percent of bowel elimination comes from bacteria. These bacteria, inhabiting the colon, feed well on and multiply better from green, leafy foods and whole grains. Good evidence of this phenomenon is discovered by an examination of stools of cows and horses living on natural green grasses. Honey, especially in the comb, also promotes these bacteria.

For many readers, this question immediately comes to mind: Where did these bacteria originate?

The origin of the colon bacteria (flora) begins from the wonderful colostrum of the mother's milk. During pregnancy, this colostrum remains stored in the nipple for the new life. As soon as the baby is born, it is important that the baby begin nursing right away. This nursing eventually implants colostrum into the baby's colon where it begins to multiply, living perpetually on the colon wall. This flora is of utmost value because it immunizes the baby against disease and will continue to do so as long as that person eats enough raw foods.

Perhaps, by now, you begin to understand why I link most body problems to the colon—to some degree. And most diseases and abnormalities, discussed in the following chapters, almost always lead us to the colon as one major problem and source of difficulty.

THE CASE OF TIM HAMMOND

A defective, poorly operating colon can cause headache. A few years ago, I made a house call to see a small boy in Chandler, Indiana, suffering excruciating headaches. He had undergone extensive medical examinations and hospital tests but had been released because doctors could find no cause for this pain.

As I examined him, I checked his rectum and found it packed full of hard fecal matter. Immediately, I began to clean him with enemas while at his home and, later, with colonic irrigations at my clinic. The boy's headaches soon disappeared, and we have become friends. From that point on, when the boy had any problems, his mother would bring him to our clinic.

Today this young man is an excellent physical specimen—all because he learned early that his diet determined his health. Recently (November 1, 1983) he wrote me the following:

I'm in track, throwing shot-put and discus. I'm also in body-building and I'm in love with my music even more than before. I also like tennis, swimming, and racquetball a lot. In general, I love sports and the competition that comes with them.

At our clinic, we taught him (as we teach all our patients) what to eat to produce a healthy colon—a diet of nature's foods, raw foods, plenty of bulk and fiber, leafy green vegetables, and whole grains. He learned that at times he needed more laxative foods, such as young greens, corn, asparagus, rhubarb, okra, parsley, berries, melons, raw nuts, and certain raw and dried fruits. We also taught him to care for and to maintain his whole body, as we intend to show you. In the following chapters on specific diseases and problems of the body, I will teach you, dear reader—as I taught him—a philosophy and methods of healing.

CLOSING COMMENT

Practically any condition of the body, if caught in time, can be regenerated by the blood, as long as the person possesses willingness, determination, and assurance that healing can result.

Let us consider, for example, the condition of hemorrhoids and varicose veins. By understanding the original cause, we merely reverse the process to heal. Since both disorders are caused partially by the body's demineralized condition, then it only stands to reason that the body needs more minerals. Another cause of these two conditions is pressure from abdominal organs, and an overloaded condition of the liver. Such pressures may be the effect of fat (obesity), pregnancy, poor posture, straining, or stress. All of these, however, rank as secondary factors to the primary state of deficiency.

Blood must be fed properly if cells function properly. Abnormal growth of the cell produces cancers and polyps (for further discussion, see chapter on "Cancer").

Yet having said these things about the body possessing potential to heal itself—provided it receives the natural resources the blood requires to heal—the person also must be determined to become well and to know he can do so.

Note: Because of necessary book-length limitations, I describe briefly the fore-going ideas of mine; but in my practice they have become most important. For the person desiring a more complete discussion of the colon and its relationship to good health, I recommend *Colon Health* by Norman W. Walker, D.Sc., Ph.D.

Chapter VI

CROHN'S DISEASE

Crohn's Disease, named after B. B. Crohn who helped to classify the complex symptoms, is a condition that previously began typically about age twenty-five. Today, however, I see more and more cases occurring in the mid-teens. Crohn's Disease (or Ileitis) refers to inflammation of the ileum. Regional Ileitis (Crohn's Disease) refers to a condition of (apparent) inflammation of an area of the small intestine, accompanied by colic-like abdominal pain, irregularity of bowels, loss of weight, and slight fever. The abdomen distends, and the victim feels thickened intestines. The narrowed intestinal canal may become obstructed, necessitating immediate surgery.

Strange as it may seem, I remember now how over the years the same symptoms were mine and my disease was diagnosed as Colitis or Ileitis and doctors told me I would have to live with it! Time, however, taught me that pure, fresh, poison-free food gradually would liberate me from the many related problems—as I also learned from my patients' recoveries.

THE CASE OF JILL

In January 1982, a sixteen-year-old lady, five-feet tall, and weighing only ninety pounds was brought to our clinic. After spending the last four years in and out of the hospital, and spending more time in bed than in school the fourth year, Jill was fed-up with doctors and didn't care if she lived or died. She was paranoid, had considered suicide, and constantly felt so bad that it was an effort for her to get out of bed many mornings.

SYMPTOMS, BEHAVIOR, TREATMENTS
A few months earlier, after suffering nausea, diarrhea, and stomach pains for four years, Jill had spent one month in a clinic out of state where they diagnosed her condition as Crohn's Disease. At that clinic, she received Prednisone to control bowel inflammation, which helped to increase her appetite and gave her more energy. At this time, she weighed only 65 pounds, not much for someone five-feet tall.

After coming home, Jill was taken off the Prednisone and began to gain weight. But before long, the pain and discomfort she had experienced returned; she became disoriented and couldn't concentrate; her medications lost their effectiveness; and as her diarrhea returned, she again lost weight and continued to worsen.

During her childhood, Jill had no noticeable problems until she was four years old when she began to suffer recurring ear infections. When five, she was diagnosed as having viral meningitis, and was given IV's. From then to her teens, she suffered from allergies, with head and chest congestion. During her ninth year, after a second testing for allergies, her doctor confirmed that she was allergic to several things and administered allergy shots which resulted in soreness, swelling, and fever in her arm from these shots.

The next three years, Jill gradually was taken off shots and medications as her symptoms diminished, but by age twelve, she began to suffer more problems. She began to suffer from diarrhea, nausea, and inability to keep food on her stomach. As food odors made her sick, she wouldn't eat and began to lose weight. She would come home from school, sleep all afternoon, try to eat supper, and then go back to bed. During her thirteenth year, she was admitted to the hospital where she underwent extensive tests and x-rays.

Between thirteen and sixteen, Jill was in and out of the hospital as she continued to experience nausea and diarrhea, frequently accompanied by chronic cramps and abdominal pain. Sometimes during four to five days at a time, she hurt so badly that she could not stand to be touched, and remained in bed. When she did feel like being up, she could eat four and five large meals a day but would continue to lose weight. One physician suggested that all her problems might be emotional.

OUR CLINIC TREATMENT FOR JILL

Upon recommendation of close church friends, in January 1982, Jill's parents brought her to our clinic. During a thorough examination, I discovered ulcers in her bowels and other Crohn-related problems. Immediately she was taken off all her previous medications and steroids, and her treatment was begun. This treatment consisted of heat packs to her back and abdominal area, softening enemas, colonics, osteopathic manipulation, degravitation with a backswing, a diet plan of kelp, protomorphogens (nucleo protein extract from a raw gland or tissue of beef excluding the fat), honey and bee pollen, colon cleansers, bentonite, raw salads and juices, and eventually fish and chicken. In her fourth month of treatment, Jill began to realize that she was getting better and would live a full, normal life again. By May, she rapidly began to improve, experienced minor pain, had increased spurts of energy, and was amazed at her improvement.

Today, one year later, Jill comes to our clinic only once every other month and is an active and vivacious student participating in her school's drama program and other activities. She still continues her natural diet and finds that she seldom craves or desires the junk foods she once enjoyed.

Jill has learned through her own experience about the totality of life and health and how the body's physical health determines the mind's health. She came to us expecting pills and shots and discovered that her treatment was nutrition, structural correction, and time. It is difficult, especially for a young person, to understand that there is no one magic cure. Jill had to learn that since her condition resulted from years of degeneration, it,

Crohn's Disease

likewise, may require years for her body to heal and regenerate. Most patients with Crohn's Disease can reflect over their past and recognize those years of degeneration.

THE CASE OF LYNN

Another patient, Lynn Hathaway, suffered her first colon attack at age twelve. Eight years later, doctors diagnosed her second attack as appendicitis. After her doctor removed her appendix, he confessed that her problem actually lay in her colon. A few years later, an Indianapolis specialist informed her that she had Crohn's Disease.

Lynn came to our clinic several months after her worst, almost fatal attack. She had first become ill in January with vomiting and diarrhea, thought to be influenza. Within the next two months, she had 20-35 bowel movements daily and began losing weight. Her weight dropped from 135 to 89 pounds between April and July, when she first arrived at our clinic. Her doctor prescribed a medicine over the phone to stop the diarrhea; this medicine worsened her condition. By April, with Lynn still suffering from the same symptoms, her doctor told her she needed a good rest. While Lynn vacationed in Florida, a nutritionist counseled her and placed her on milk products and assorted vitamins. Both symptoms and weight loss continued: Lynn eventually wound up in an Indianapolis hospital, where she received cortisone. After two weeks and negligible change, she was released and sent home to recuperate. Lynn began to have black-out spells, however, and eventually went into a convulsion. After one week in her hometown hospital, she returned home and continued to worsen. When friends began to notice a green discoloration in her skin, they insisted on bringing her to our clinic. Today, she remembers her first week here—how she suffered such pain that she could not bear to feel her undergarments and bed linens against her skin. She remembers wishing that she could die soon.

After two weeks of treatment and proper diet, however, Lynn began to realize she felt better, and began her path to recovery. Today she exemplifies good health and displays abundant optimism about her future. And Lynn, like Jill, has led a full, industrious, and relatively pain-free life as she assists her body in its healing.

And this treatment is true for hundreds of our patients, as we witness the general pattern: recurring symptoms, irrelevant medical treatment, worsening condition—then, regeneration toward health following our clinic's treatments.

THE CASE OF ANDY

As you have seen in the cases discussed, it is possible to regenerate the colon. As the colon revives, it attempts to regain its normal shape. The patient also comes back to life. Andy Jessee, confined to his bed not too long ago, now lifts weights, has graduated from his high school, and holds a part-time job. He also was diagnosed as having Crohn's Disease.

ANDY'S PREVIOUS PROBLEMS

Andy's problems began in eighth grade with a duodenal ulcer which later developed into intestinal inflammation. The cramps and pain in the abdomen occurred intermittently but regularly. He received Tetracycline and a sulfa drug to coat his stomach. At age seventeen, he had eighteen inches of small and large intestines removed. Six months after surgery, Andy developed the flu and received Amoxil. Before long, he developed diarrhea, cramping, loss of appetite, and began losing weight. This time he received Prednisone and a sulfa drug.

OUR CLINIC'S TREATMENT FOR ANDY

When Andy came to our clinic in July 1981, he had spent much of his school year in bed, suffering with pains he was convinced would remain with him the rest of his life. But after his second day of treatment, he began to feel relief in his abdomen, and before many more days he felt better all over. Andy was taken off drugs and medication several months prior to treatment at our clinic, and treated much the same as other patients with Crohn's.

This procedure is the general treatment plan: After initial examination, we first concentrate on cleansing the bowel. We cleanse with various types of enemas and colonic irrigations and use of "Natural Relief" (montmorillonite) and "Veico" (bentonite). Next, we utilize necessary forms of bulk to sweep the colon and stimulate the colon wall muscle to contract: these bulks include ground psyllium seed, a sea vegetation called "Sea Klenze," "Coloklenz" (produced by V.E. Irons Co.) and other bulks which cause this physical action. The patient is encouraged to drink fresh fruit and vegetable juices, pure water and huniger (vinegar and honey in water) each day, and to change the diet entirely to raw foods such as fruits, vegetable, nuts, melons, and berries. Besides the patient's needing these foods for fiber content, we teach the patient that the quality of food is directly proportionate to the quality of blood or vice versa and consequently to each part of the patient's body. We also employ mineral and vitamin supplements to help build quality blood and glandular substances called protomorphogens. These latter substances promote rejuvenation of each endocrine organ. Heat packs are applied to stomach and back area to reduce pain and encourage healing. When the patient is able, osteopathic manipulative treatment is administered to stimulate the body's healing processes. Sinuses are examined, and necessary structural corrections are instituted—along with use of the suction. The usual needed structural changes occur in the nose, post nasal area, tonsils, and the trachea—not neglecting the facial bones and bones of the mouth and the teeth.

This treatment for Crohn's also is used for most all colon diseases such as colitis, diverticulitis and diverticulosis; obstruction of the colon such as benign or cancerous tumors within, around, or inside the wall of the colon; or volvulus (a twisted or looped area of the intestine).

Crohn's Disease

Besides degeneration of colon tissue and muscle, many colon problems are increased by its deformation. Practically all colons today are deformed, (ptosed, fallen, hanging down from proper position). This deformation results from degeneration caused by a diet of demineralized foods over the years. As these foods are consumed continously, the colon wall muscle degenerates and deteriorates, resulting in weak and flabby walls. The colon no longer possesses the muscle tone to keep it strong and to hold its normal shape; so it stretches, lengthens, and loops. In this process, the colon resembles blowing up a balloon. The new balloon will be firm and strong, but once it has been blown up and stretched, it then becomes flabby and atonic.

So you see, there exist many causes for these colon abnormalities, but if we first understand them, then treatment is simply to eliminate that cause and assist nature as it attempts to heal. Proper treatment can restore colon health—a key to body health.

Chapter VII

EAR, NOSE, AND THROAT

Today's cold medicines and remedies are advertised to "ease the pain and discomfort of the cold or cold symptoms"; but you will notice, however, advertisers are wise enough never to suggest that the remedy will cure colds. Dictionaries explain that the term "remedy" means cure, restorative, counter-action, reparation, relief, aid, help, and assistance. Actually, then, today's cold remedies merely offer relief, not cure. Recently, I heard an allergist speaking at a medical convention state that the most he could hope to attain for allergies was relief, implying that a cure (total remission) is impossible. This assertion would lead one to believe that colds are inherent and allergies are permanent, which is *not* true.

Everyone seeks a cure for the common cold. There are promises of financial rewards for the first person to cure the common cold. If this great break-through—a cure—ever occurs, it will result in irreparable after-effects, assuming that 'cure' means eliminating symptoms of a cold. Our goal should be to eliminate the cause or causes of the cold, resulting in *no need* for the cold (nor a cure).

THE COMMON COLD: A NATURAL LAW

The cold is another of God's natural laws in action. It demonstrates a natural law operating in the body. Body responses are tremendously good and necessary to promote life. It is necessary for the body to exhibit a *cold* as it is necessary for your car to speed if you accelerate with your foot pedal and expect your speed to increase.

Animals living out-of-doors do not show signs of runny noses and sore throats, unless we have fed them unnatural, highly-cooked, refined, and devitalized foods. Many doctors and scientists now accept that there are mucous-forming foods. Doctors tell most asthma sufferers that they are "allergic to all milk and wheat products." I say this *allergy* is the body's action or reaction as it attempts to eliminate toxins resulting from undigested foods, dead foods, unnatural additives and chemicals on our foods, poisons we breathe (e.g., air pollution), and unnatural creams and lotions applied to and absorbed by our skins, etc. Any element not in its *natural state* (which the body was designed to act upon and utilize) becomes a toxin for the body to eliminate, and formation of mucous functions as part of that elimination system.

THE NOSE: ADHESIONS

Various reasons account for this "cold response," usually first noticed as a "runny nose." The nose was designed to warm and cool the air, to moisten or dry the air, and to filter foreign bodies as air enters the body. To accomplish all of these, it is necessary that a person breathe well and thoroughly through the nose. Equally essential, spaces within the nose must remain open, unobstructed. In all my years of practice, I have never seen a normal nose; I believe that every one needs to normalize his nose structure to some extent. Common colds, allergies, constant sneezing as in the case of hay fever, a hacking cough, or inability to breathe properly are evidence of obstructions in the nose. The sneeze is the body's antagonistic movement to eliminate an overload. Pollen is offensive, causing sneezing or excessive secretion, because the filters (turbinates) are swollen and cannot filter the air properly. The most common obstructions include swelling, adhesions, and polyps. One or more of these conditions occur in most civilized peoples.

The most frequent obstruction, swelling, often results from mucous-forming foods (refined sugars and grains, milk products, overly-cooked foods, and highly processed foods). Continued use of these foods overloads the blood and the lymph; as a result, the filters (turbinates) swell from the overload. Whenever constant swelling occurs in the nose, the same swelling problem almost always will be present in the bowel.

When a nose is swollen consistently—even occasionally for only a few hours at one period—adhesions will form where one membrane touches another. These adhesions, much like cobwebs, form over a period of time. They develop around and between surfaces of the turbinates, septum, and lateral outer wall. These adhesions develop as the lymph, a collagenous material, is converted into connective tissue for the purpose of reinforcement during the healing process, which requires inflammation or swelling. Therefore, we are justified in breaking or removing adhesions after the healing process has occurred and the connective tissue is needed no longer.

Before we proceed with our discussion of the nose, a few definitions may help. The septum is a wall separating two cavities or masses of softer substance or tissue, and the turbinate is a thin, plicated, bony or cartilaginous plate covered with olfactory and mucous membrane borne on the walls of the nasal chambers. Three turbinates project from the nose's outer (lateral) wall. (See Figure 7) By location, the middle turbinate is the most vulnerable of the three because of its relationship to sinus openings or exits.

Adhesions begin to form as soon as a person begins eating refined, devitalized foods, beginning in earliest infancy with babies on man-made formula, and can remain a lifetime.

When adhesions occur around the middle turbinate, they obstruct ventilation to and drainage from the sinuses. Exactly as scar tissues do, adhesions will shorten as they age, worsening the obstruction. The

Ear, Nose, and Throat

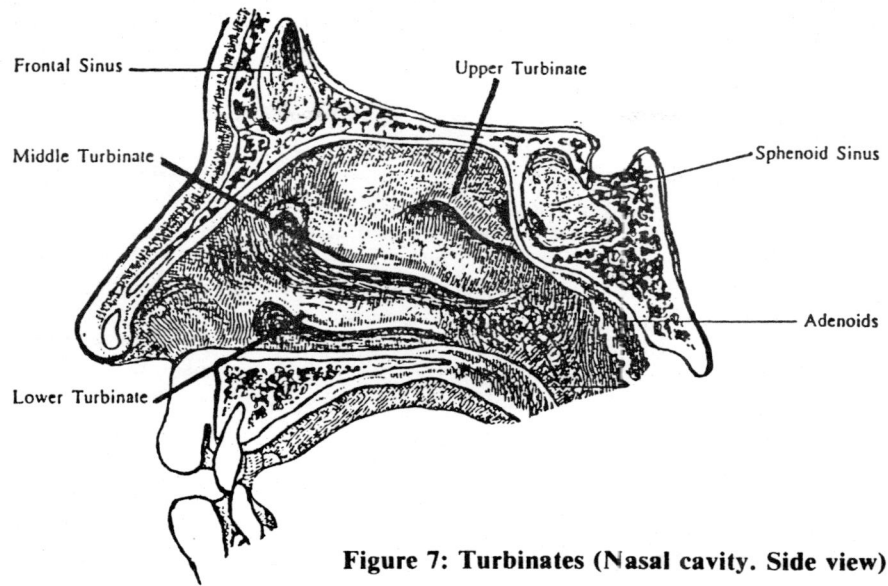

Figure 7: Turbinates (Nasal cavity. Side view)

turbinates, which normally hang downward, are pulled down even more by these shortening adhesions. As a result, a person's sinus problems continue to worsen until corrected. Ventilation, necessary to permit air into the sinuses, is prevented from doing so when the turbinate (filter) is pulled down over the opening of the sinus, also the air exit.

CORRECTION OF NASAL ADHESIONS

Step One. Correction of these adhesions in the nose is done, first, by deadening the area with a topical anesthetic (the anesthetic applied to the surface is picked up by the mucous membrane). Then, when the turbinates are deadened sufficiently, the operator uses a flat instrument to break the adhesions, eventually breaking loose and freeing the turbinate. This treatment is frequently necessary for a month or more to prevent the turbinate from growing back together where it abnormally adhered.

Step Two. The next step goes beyond the nose and corrects adhesions formed in the post nasal space (also called nasopharynx), an area beyond the palate and behind the nose at the beginning of the eustachian tubes, and corrects adhesions formed in the eustachian tubes to the middle ears. This procedure includes adhesions in and around the adenoids. This procedure must be executed digitally, or by the finger (seeing with the finger) as it can only be done poorly with an instrument. The operator carefully feels for adhesions and/or enlarged glands—excessive glands of lymphatic tissue formed to facilitate elimination of waste. These can be broken down conveniently and thereby eliminated except for a necessary amount of adenoid or other tonsil tissue imperatively always needed. Most adhesions can be removed by this conservative osteopathic finger surgery, so-called because it first was used and described by the osteopathic physician who performed it.

THE NOSE: POLYPS AND THEIR CORRECTION

Another common obstruction in the nose is polyps, occurring also in the sinuses (Figure 8). When a person's diet is saturated with mucous-forming foods, secretion glands in the nose and sinuses enlarge from overloading with mucous. This condition eventually will cause polyps to form—tumors, usually with a narrow base, caused by hypertrophy (overgrowth) of the nose's mucous membrane. It has been suggested that perhaps nature may have created the polyps there to increase the nose's functioning surface. Many polyps are visible to the specialist or physician; however, they may be hidden within the sinus cavities or by deformity of the nose interior.

Visible obstructing polyps can be removed conservatively in a chair at the clinic, not requiring hospitalization. Those with a pedicle (polyps with stems), and accessible with a nasal snare, a wire-lipped instrument that snips off polyps, can be removed by an operator using this snare. Those polyps not accessible in this manner can be removed by electric cautery or by some chemical destructive to the polyp.

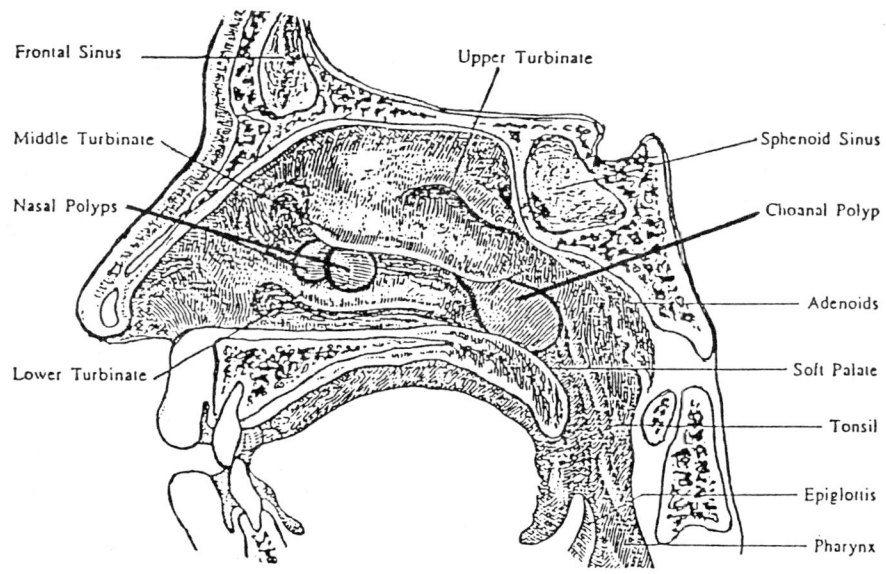

Figure 8: Polyps (Nasal cavity. Side view)

Ear, Nose, and Throat

THE EAR

At this time, 1983, health statistics indicate the existence of more than thirty million cases of deafness in America, and, no doubt, millions more have lost part of their hearing. In any public gathering today, you will notice persons wearing hearing devices and may even notice your friends asking you to repeat what you have said. Even TV programs have interpreters or "closed captions for the hearing impaired."

This situation is most commonly loss of hearing by obstruction, a blockage of the eustachian tube (See Figure 9). This blockage may result from what has been described earlier concerning adhesions. Furthermore, many cases also have involved nerve loss, caused from nerve degeneration as a result of faulty nutrition and body toxins.

When a sound wave enters your head, it must enter through the outer ear and skull and exit through the eustachian tube, nose, or mouth. If the tube is closed from swelling and/or adhesions, sound can enter the ear, but cannot exit totally. This condition causes a piling of sound vibrations or sound waves in the hearing apparatus in the middle ear and inner ear (the third ear), which makes sounds confusing, occurring in most people as they begin to deafen. Much deafness results from this obstruction and can be corrected.

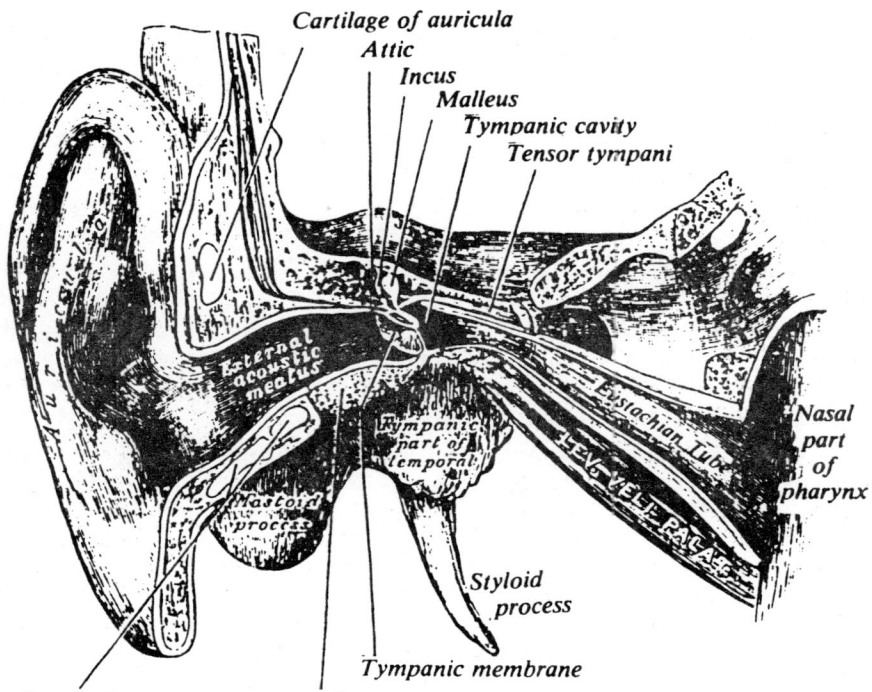

Figure 9: External and middle ear, opened anteriorly. (Right side)

CORRECTION OF AURAL ADHESIONS

The obstructive form of deafness can be eliminated partially and often totally through opening the eustachian tubes by removing adhesions as described. Nerve loss can be corrected partially and sometimes totally by a gradual process of remineralizing the body, detoxifying the body, and correcting structural faults.

Nine of ten times, even nerve deafness will respond after correcting the cause of the obstructive—partial or total closure of the eustachian tube—deafness. This corrective procedure is done by gradually dilating the opening into the eustachian tube, which must be done with the finger (for the purpose of feel). This dilation can be performed as far as the bony structure of the skull, one-half inch or more of the soft part of the eustachian tube. From there on in, the work of the bony part of the eustachian tube has to be done by kneading with the finger the muscles lining the soft part of the tube. This step also must be done gradually, since each treatment is predicated on the one before (depending on how much is accomplished with each treatment).

A frequently overlooked condition should be described here. In nearly all cases of obstructive deafness, we observe some involvement of the lower jaw. I refer to the common condition of an overbite resulting from a partially dislocated mandible. When this dislocation is restored to the normal position by a dentist skilled in bite correction, possibilities of improved hearing will increase considerably. And let me mention again that no matter how substantial the structural change, if diet is not corrected to a wholesome mucousless diet, this condition almost inevitably will return.

LYMPH, SINUSES, SECRETION, AND ELIMINATION

This conservative ear, nose, and throat surgery was taught to me after my formal training, since I had heard little of it in the osteopathic college I attended. After my graduation, and because of my own personal sinus problems, I consulted Doctor C. Paul Snyder (Philadelphia, Pennsylvania) who taught this conservative surgery because of his interest in the problems of his family.

At first I went to him as a patient but soon became his student. I remained under his training for about ten years; the first two years, I traveled back and forth every three or four months, for two weeks' training each time. Later, I returned periodically, for more courses consisting of two weeks' training. So far as I know, no one teaches this work now, and no formal teaching of it has occurred in any college. Today, doctors could train one week a month for one year to become proficient and qualified in this form of conservative eye, ear, nose, and throat treatment.

I now use this approach daily and consider it invaluable in eliminating sinus problems. Unfortunately, removing polyps and correcting adhesions is not always the only solution for sinus problems although they directly link to the excessive mucous problem.

Every sinus is lined by secretion glands to secrete juices normally to lubricate, moisten, and protect the membranes of the nose, chest, and throat. These sinuses drain naturally through action of the cilia, microscopic hairs lining the walls and belonging to the sinus gland system. These cilia wave the secretions in one direction, toward the outlet of the sinus, just as wind blowing grass. If these cilia are obstructed, they lose their function; but as the obstruction is corrected, the cilia gradually will rejuvenate and regain their function of ciliary motion.

When sinuses cannot empty freely by using obstructed and poorly functioning cilia, then secretions will pile up in the sinus. When secretions, which normally moisten and lubricate, cannot leave the sinus cavity because of obstructions, they remain in the body heat, spoil, and become waste for the body to eliminate. This elimination must be done partially by the lymph system, the avenue of escape or agent for removing waste and debris from the body. Lymph is a weak alkaline, nearly colorless coagulable fluid, contained in the lymphatic vessels. It contains colorless corpuscles, but is free from red corpuscles. Lymph may be regarded as consisting chiefly of blood plasma exuded from the blood capillaries in the various tissues and organs, and taken up by the lymphatic vessels to be discharged finally by the thoracic and right lymphatic ducts into the great veins near the heart during inflammation of some body part. It is a fibrinous material exuded from the blood vessels. In the process of healing, it is either absorbed or converted into connective tissue binding the inflamed surfaces together (connective tissue, adhesions, and fibrous tissues - all similar).

To state it simply, when the stagnant mucous in the sinus is not eliminated through the nose and throat exits, then the spoiled, toxic matter is absorbed through the sinus membrane, first passing through the lymph surrounding the cell and into the cell. It is transported then through the lymph system, back to one of the major arteries of the heart, where it is dumped back into the circulation system to be eliminated. A doctor trained with an understanding of the head can feel of the neck and tell which sinuses are obstructed the most. The problem in the front sinuses will usually be felt in the front part of the lateral side of the neck. Obstructions in the middle ear and the mastoid are usually felt behind the middle portion of the lateral wall of the neck.

The debris carried by the lymph, eventually passing through the kidneys and liver, can become a major cause of pain and discomfort of these organs and can even create crises with some destruction. The kidneys and bowel reflect stagnation in the body. Many infections eventually will wind up or show up in urine, bowel, or in air exhaled (as in "bad breath").

Dandruff also reflects waste eliminated by the body. As the scalp's secreting glands become overburdened with toxins, their abnormal composition becomes noticeable in the form of dandruff. Cooked grain products commonly cause dandruff, but this condition can be improved by using only freshly-ground grains.

All bodily respiratory membranes—ears, nose, throat, lungs, and skin—become accessory organs of elimination if the bowel is overloaded with waste. The skin's indications are pimples, skin blemishes, enlarged blood vessels, itching, irritation, psoriasis, eczema, coated tongue, etc.

Excessive mucous in the head also suggests retarded movement of body waste through the colon. This waste spoils while it remains in the body's heat, and the waste is picked up again by the lymph—resulting in overloaded mucous secretions, since the sinuses are accessory organs of elimination. An overloaded nose strongly indicates that the colon waste is retarded in its elimination.

Nearly all cases of colitis evidence sinus drainage through the digestive and eliminative systems. The colon reflects what is going on in the head—ears, nose, and throat. All patients with Crohn's Disease which I have examined also suffer from sinus problems, confirming this relationship.

As you may now see, the system links together. A doctor should be able to look into the nose to see what is going on in the colon, and, likewise, should be able to look into the colon and discover what is going on in the head. Polyps in either the nose or bowel usually reveal the same problem in the other body part. This fact was demonstrated to me more than a decade ago in a patient from Greenville, South Carolina.

THE CASE OF FRANCES

Frances Potts came to our office at the urging of our mutual Christian friend, Brother Joe Carroll, an Australian missionary. By the time she arrived at my clinic, she was so ill, depressed, and tired of living that she thought she would never be any better. Frances was, by then, exasperated with doctors; only because she trusted Brother Carroll, she decided to visit our clinic.

I learned from her, years later, that she totally trusted and confided in me only after I had examined and described the conditions of her nose to her. She told me initially she began to possess doubts about me when I explained to her that although I knew she had come to me with colon troubles, I wanted to examine her head also. I went on to explain to her that the sinus area was the upper end of the sewer, and most often sinus conditions will reflect colon conditions. Frances had not told me that doctors had been removing polyps from her rectal area periodically for some time. When I discovered that the whole left side of her nose was closed with a polyp, and told her so, her doubts disappeared, and she decided to go along totally with my treatment. She went on a program of colonics: heat packs to her back and abdominal areas; osteopathic manipulation; a diet of raw grapes, fruit juices, and huniger (See Glossary.) As her nausea diminished, she was able to eat fruit salads and eventually vegetable salads. Finally, the polyp was

Ear, Nose, and Throat

removed from her nose, and she could lay her head on a pillow and breathe again, which she said she had not been able to do for as long as she could remember. Because she had so much to overcome, Frances needed almost two weeks to begin to feel any better.

As a weak and frail child, Frances would become ill with nausea and vomiting at the beginning of her summers when she began playing in the sun. During her early years, she often experienced hard stomach cramps and chronic constipation and remembers how hard it was to get up in the mornings and dress herself, which continued through her twenties.

Because of leg and feet pains at age 34, Frances was examined and told that her uterus was tilted and needed to be removed, which was soon done along with the removal of her appendix. In her late 30's, still having the same problems, she began to suffer much rectal bleeding. Because of increasing pain, she spent a good portion of each day in bed. Medications and sitz baths were prescribed, but finally she was given a hemorrhoidectomy. During her second hemorrhoidectomy, a rectal fistula was discovered and removed. One year later, Frances had a hiatal hernia operation. During these years, as a result of the tranquilizers, nerve pills, antibiotics, and pain killers she was receiving constantly, Frances was often puffy, swollen, lethargic.

When Frances came to me, at age 45, she was so drained that each day she awoke, she felt worse than the day before. As we mentioned, Frances needed two weeks to begin to overcome all the medications she had been taking (she had discontinued them the first day at our clinic). The beginning of the third week, she noticed significant improvements: Her pain was easing, her nausea was almost gone, and she was able to eat a much greater variety of fruits and vegetables. By the end of the third week, she was a different person. According to Frances, "When I came home, I could see better; my eyes had improved so much that I no longer had to read with a magnifying glass; my mind cleared; I had a new sense of life; and the whole world had taken on a new meaning for me." She was so enthusiastic about learning to heal herself and to keep herself well that she could not wait to spread the word. Frances began working part-time in a natural food store nearby, and spent spare hours teaching others of health and nutrition. Today Frances is still a bundle of energy, although now in her late 60's. She told me recently that the best years of her life followed her visits to our clinic.

But Frances' case is not the first nor the last since every day each case over the years has proven to me the idea of the dynamic interrelated totality of the body and life itself. This idea was understood and accepted, by record, in the early Christian era. In I Corinthians 12:12-30, writing to members of the early church in Corinth, Paul related the totality and interdependence of the body's parts—the dependence of each part upon the other and the individual importance of each member in its relationship to the whole—to the totality and interdependence of the new church's members, emphasizing each member's importance to each other and to the whole church.

TONSILS, ADENOIDS, AND SECRETION

Because the body was designed to work as a whole, it is unrealistic to believe it will function one-hundred-percent with certain parts removed. Thank goodness, today, we are not so ready to remove tonsils and adenoids as in the past, since evidently tonsils and adenoids are essential to health.

These structures are a part of the protective mechanism of the body and are lymphoid tissue. They do not need to be removed! Frequently, either or both may become swollen and/or loaded with adhesions, interfering with their normal functions. All that is necessary to normalize them is to remove the adhesions and eliminate the cause of the swelling. It is *not* necessary to remove them surgically. This ring of tonsil tissue in the throat is one of the body's first lines of defense. There nature provided so much machinery to neutralize poison before it passes beyond.

Tonsils and adenoids, located on the back wall of the nasopharynx, secrete and excrete. Juices they secrete lubricate, bathe the throat, and keep it healthy. They excrete to eliminate as they overload with debris.

The tonsil, formed more or less like a strawberry, has crypts which increase its surface area to engulf waste dripping or running from the sinuses, over the adenoid and the tonsils. As these tonsils overload constantly with stagnant secretion, they swell and develop adhesions in their crypts. Adhesions must then be broken loose within the crypts. This procedure is done with a blunt ball-point instrument, and often requires many treatments, since there are dozens of crypts. Visible crypts are worked on. As tonsils are cleaned out and the person's diet corrected, these tonsils again will be able to fulfill their occupation of absorbing the toxins while neutralizing the toxic material, excreting waste, and engaging in production of new blood and lymph components. As explained, it is normal for the sinus secretions to drain backward and down the throat, but it is when these secretions are stagnant that they create a sore throat by denuding or eroding the throat's otherwise normal membrane. A swollen throat also can be caused by overloaded lymph, as the blood constantly and fervantly attempts to pick up stagnant secretion. The body demonstrates its activity of trying to eliminate a poison that would eventually wind up in the stomach if it weren't absorbed by the lymph and blood.

When this stagnant secretion does wind up in the stomach, it interferes with digestion and elimination. Because it is a false food, a toxin, the body attempts to handle it through digestion, elimination, and assimilation. The toxic part must be eliminated as a poison, irritating the bowel, kidneys, and bladder.

Swelling will disappear in the throat after shrinking the nose, using suction to drain the sinuses as much as possible, and correcting the diet. This nose suction, performed by a vacuum-type machine, is invaluable in clearing the sinuses. I use it anytime I perform ear, nose, and throat treatment.

Ear, Nose, and Throat

DEVIATION OF THE MIDDLE PARTITION AND ITS CORRECTION

Nearly every Caucasion possesses a deviation of the middle partition (the septum) of the nose. Most such deviations can be corrected by anesthetizing the area and repeatedly breaking down the septum with the little finger or a flat metal instrument. As the septum breaks down, it also realigns so that it no longer obstructs the normal passage. After the nose is normalized, to permit the sinuses to drain properly as they were intended to do, it is usually necessary to continue to use the suction to draw the remaining residue from the sinuses. This procedure must be conducted over a period of time, since the stagnant mucous will contain old debris and cheesy material formed from juices retained in the sinuses through the years. These materials were formed from the time the nasal obstructions began forming. These juices having remained in the sinuses too long, allowed the solid part to settle in the bottom of the cavity, where it became solid and cheesy as it aged. The liquid part—the supernatent fluid (liquid part of the secretion)—would rise and drain through the nose or throat. As a proper mucousless diet is incorporated, as the blood condition improves, and as structural problems are corrected, the body will begin to liquify the cheesy material so that it can be eliminated normally with the use of suction and ciliary motion.

Not long ago, a four-year-old girl who was losing her hearing came to our clinic. Her mother had noticed that the child could not hear her unless standing face to face with the child, and the child watched her talk. Her family physician told her not to worry—that it was only a cold, and placed the child on antibiotics. After shrinking the little girl's nose, I removed one-half teacupful of thick mucous from her nose and sinuses. The mother was amazed that the child's hearing improved immediately, amazed enough now to enjoy a healthy child on a near mucousless diet, free from colds.

SOME EYE AILMENTS AND THEIR CORRECTION

Many common eye ailments occur because the conjunctiva, the membrane lining the eyelid's inner surface and reflected over the eyeball's fore part, cannot drain through its normal exit, which may be plugged by problems or obstructions in the nose. The eye's normal flow drains under the middle turbinate in the nose. These turbinates act as radiators, dehumidifiers, and humidifiers. Their cartilage, covered by mucous membrane, runs the length of the nose, from front to rear, protruding from the side wall of the nose into the nose (See Figure 7). From this picture, we can see why excessive snoring can indicate some form of obstruction in the head. The middle turbinate covers most of the sinuses' exits, and these exits can be loosened to clear the obstruction by removal of adhesions. After completing this procedure, I attempt to shrink the nose by applying, with a cotton tip applicator, an anesthetic to the turbinates. When the turbinates are reduced sufficiently, I use a suction to pull as much secretion out of the sinuses as will come, by suctioning the opening of the nasal lacrimal ducts, the duct from the eye to the nose (See Figure 10).

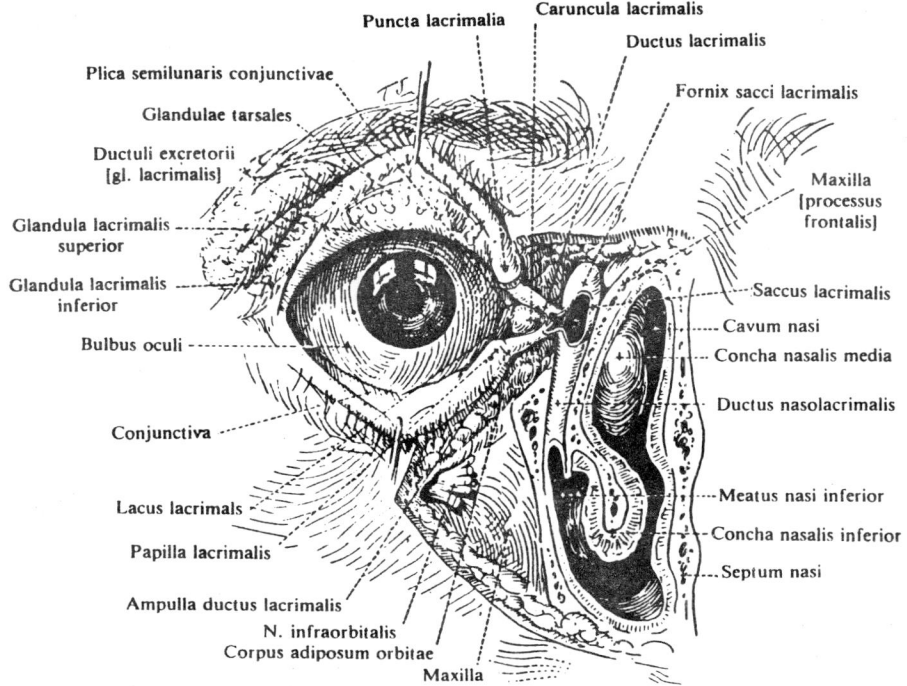

Figure 10: Topography of the lacrimal apparatus.

When this duct is obstructed, secretions will back up into the eye, causing frequent eye overflow. Chalazion, a cyst of the lid, results from this chronic blockage of eye duct drainage. A cyst only results from accumulation of fluid in an obstructed gland. Styes simply result from overloading the eye's normal secretion and from faulty secretion composition.

Glaucoma also can be handled successfully by using these same principles and approach to eye, ear, nose, and throat. But remember, even with all the structural corrections, the diet must be corrected. Mucous-forming foods must be eliminated. With all the unnatural elements human beings are exposed to—pollutants, toxins, additives, synthetics, artificial chemicals, processed and refined foods—we need maximum nutrition and assimilation to aid the body as it attempts to process and eliminate them.

TUBERCULOSIS

My dad, also an osteopath, who died at 61 from heart disease, was never healthy. His family had always kept a cow; thus, he was raised on milk products. He constantly had mucous drainage, sinus trouble, and puss. In his mid-teens, he was told he had consumption (now termed tuberculosis).

Ear, Nose, and Throat

Tuberculosis is caused from degeneration resulting from over-cooking of foods and too many mucous-forming foods. Rice is highly mucous-forming. Similar to leprosy, tuberculosis results from lack of necessary mineral elements and mucous overload which occurs commonly among rice-eating people (See *The Mucousless Diet* by Arnold Ehret). Cavities occur in the lungs and other organs because of this deficiency. The lung, a sponge-like structure, will begin to disintegrate, causing these cavities and spaces to form where mucous will accumulate, the reason for heavy cough. This condition can begin to heal as soon as the patient follows a raw diet, minus all refined grains and milk products. Some excellent tissue-building foods for prevention and treatment of tuberculosis include dark green vegetables, fresh fruits, raw nuts, berries, and melons. For best success, the patient should eat only a raw diet. This same diet we use when we treat any sinus problem, colds, influenza, or related problems. We also flood the patient with plenty of fluids and liquid foods, and clean out the elimination system, (as explained in the chapter on detoxifying).

A good treatment for pneumonia is a vinegar water enema every hour (one tablespoon vinegar per pint of warm water) and warm vinegar drinks (one tablespoon apple vinegar and less raw honey than vinegar per eight ounces of distilled water) before each enema, until the patient begins to improve.

The body's reaction, indicating "disease," is not the problem to be treated, but indicates the problem. We must understand why the body reacts as it does, and understand the cause of the reaction. *You* should study your own body operation. When your body overloads with toxins, its excretory glands will increase bodily secretion. Mucous is a natural secretion. These increased secretions constitute the body's added effort to mobilize stagnant waste and to remove it from the body. A cold *is always necessary when it occurs.* If we lived, however, by total natural law, our bodies inevitably would *need no cold or cold-related disease.* But since we are bombarded constantly by these toxins, we can aid the body's healing abilities only when we understand the cause and treatment of these body reactions, indicators, or "diseases."

Chapter VIII
ASTHMA AND EMPHYSEMA
ASTHMA

Asthma is a disease characterized by difficulty of breathing (because of spasmodic contraction of the bronchi) which recurs at intervals and is accompanied by a wheezing sound, a sense of chest constriction, cough, and expectoration.

This disorder in breathing makes it difficult for a person to live normally. Such a person will suffer attacks of faulty or labored breathing and may even experience short periods of inability to breathe.

Normal breathing is diaphragmatic breathing, plus some costal (within the rib cage) breathing; but in asthma, the diaphragm and rib muscles tighten, and become spastic, causing breathing to become difficult.

All asthmatics are constipated; most will suffer from spastic colon and other physical problems such as fallen abdominal organs, hardening arteries, alkalosis, and adhesions in ear, nose, and throat. The spastic colon causes blood to be so alkaline that it thickens and cannot move normally, causing the bronchi and the turbinates in the nose and lung passages to narrow and swell. These tightened vessels and tightened breathing tubes—plus the thickened blood—interfere with normal breathing, until the person experiences a paroxysm, or asthma attack.

Causes of alkalosis are the same causes of excessive mucous. Remember that mucous is a natural vehicle from mucous-forming glands in the body to *transport waste material* (to carry it off). When the body overloads with indigestible foods, foods creating greater alkalosis, pollutants from air and water, or any other unnatural element the body would need to try to eliminate, a heavy or thicker mucous will form which will not be able to travel normally. This mucous and the alkalosis promotes swelling and tightening, until asthma and/or emphysema results.

EMPHYSEMA

Actually, the underlying cause for asthma and emphysema is basically the same, merely different degrees of the same disorder. Emphysema is brought on by asthma. In emphysema, dead areas have developed in the lungs, preventing air in or out. Tobacco smoking, for example, coats the small alveolae (air sacs), until they can't fulfill their job to transmit oxygen and the gasses which return in exchange for oxygen. Asthma precedes emphysema.

Treatment for asthma and emphysema is much the same as any other disease or abnormal condition of the body. Basically, we use the same approach with regard to the three principles discussed throughout the book; toxins, nutrition, and structure correction. It is not necessary for anyone to suffer with asthma, no matter how old he is nor the number of years he has suffered.

THE CASE OF
THE REVEREND MONSIGNOR WILLIAM JARBOE

The Reverend Monsignor William B. Jarboe was seventy-three years old when doctors told him he suffered from hardening arteries and emphysema, both of which progressively would worsen, since there was no cure. Just before his forced retirement from the priesthood because of his illness, he constructed his own coffin in his basement workshop. When he came to our clinic, he suffered from emphysema so badly it totally exhausted him to walk from one room to the other; he was extremely lethargic; he had excessive mucous and shortness of breath; and his lungs contained excessive fluid.

He was given various osteopathic treatments, colonics, etc. and was placed on a mucous-free diet of no meat, breads, dairy products, starches, sugars, and he was fed soybeans for protein, honey for his sweet cravings, and raw vegetables, fruits, melons, berries, nuts, and pure water huniger.

Within two weeks, he breathed normally; by the end of two months, he dug out his basement to enlarge his workshop; and two years later he left his retirement and accepted another parish. Now, at eighty-two, he says he probably should sell his coffin before the termites eat it up. His cholestrol level is normal, and he still occasionally works in his basement workshop.

The severity of The Reverend Monsignor Jarboe's case has little to do with treatment results; if anything, it can be to the patient's advantage. The more severe the asthma, the more determined and dedicated the patient will be to treatment and diet.

Such was the case of a young patient from Indiana.

BRANDY'S CASE

Brandy Wilhite's parents brought him over when he was seven years old. Since the time Brandy was eighteen months old—when his asthma began—he had seldom slept through a night. His parents slept in shifts so they could listen to his breathing, for warning of an attack. Doctors had taken most of his toys away from him; the new ones were all non-allergenic; he could not run or go outside to play; and many of his days he spent in hospital emergency rooms under oxygen tents. The family had given up hope that he would ever be better; his mother was at school six times a day, administering his medication and checking his breathing; and the family's

Asthma and Emphysema

doctor and hospital bills were astronomical. On friends' advice, and in total desperation, they brought him to our clinic. After the tenth day of treatment and diet, Brandy began to sleep through the night, and each day he rapidly improved. Today, one year later, he leads a happy, busy normal life; plays football; and enjoys all the other sports and pleasures of his friends. His mother remains conscientious about his diet and prepares his lunches for him to carry to school. Brandy is evidence that determination and dedication of patient and family is essential to recovery.

And I emphasize here that sustained cooperation of the patient's family is essential, for—as much as doctors can do—responsibility of staying on diet and avoiding ingesting foods infested with chemicals and polluted with refined products and processes must be shared by all family members. Another patient, Kirk Boster, and his family illustrate this fact. Kirk, six years old, came to us with asthmatic problems.

KIRK'S CASE

And I want to share with you Kirk's story. In the past several pages, however, you have listened mostly to me. You will enjoy hearing from his mother the story of Kirk's battles and eventual return to good health. To record for herself this odyssey, she wrote a long letter. What follows is her letter, as she wrote it, dated August 21, 1983, and written at the family home in Fairfield, Illinois:

I stand looking down at this long-legged child asleep on the couch. I listen to his deep regular breathing and marvel how the summer sun has bleached his hair while tanning his body to golden bronze. The rhythm of his deep breathing is a song of peace. As I lift him to carry him off to bed, my heart fills with gratitude. This night we all can rest. I can go to sleep without listening in my subconscious for the sound of his labored breathing and the gripping anxieties that have plagued our days and nights for most of his lifetime.

Kirk Andrew Boster was born April 26, 1977, a healthy baby weighing 8 pounds and 13 ounces. He was welcomed into our family by two older brothers, James Paul, 8, and Frank, 2. I breast-fed Kirk for seven months. When I started back to work, his food supply dried up. He could not tolerate the formula the doctor recommended; so he was switched to goat's milk. Finally, in desperation, he was placed on jello water.

Soon after the pediatrician started him on the jello protein formula, he started suffering frequent ear infections and bronchitis. After a ten-day stint of antibiotics, he would be off perhaps two weeks, and then the infection would recur.

When Kirk was 12 months old, our pediatrician referred us to another pediatrician, a specialist in allergies. He did numerous tests and started Kirk on two allergy shots weekly. Kirk had been taking short-term doses of Prednisone, but when he was 16 months he received it daily.

At Christmas 1978, Kirk became sick, and I decided to call our family doctor instead of making the long drive to St. Louis. Our doctor was horrified when I told him Kirk was on Prednisone and had been for several months. He asked if I were aware of the side effects. I was not. I implicitly trusted the wisdom of our Pediatrician. And although I was disturbed deeply that we were not obtaining results, it didn't occur to me that we actually might be damaging the future health of this child.

We were referred to yet another specialist who said that all we could do was leave him on Prednisone. We could not accept that; so, we searched for another opinion. Kirk lay in the hospital in a croup tent for eight days (February 1979) with bronchitis. Our doctor started him on Theophyllin, and he seemed to respond. We started to St. Louis to the pediatric allergist. At two years of age, Kirk weighed only 22 pounds. He was extremely pale with dark circles under his eyes. (I had the same from lack of sleep and anxiety.)

When Kirk would have a severe attack (invariably at night), we would rush to the Emergency Room at the local hospital, and he would receive an adrenalin shot. Sometimes, he would require a second shot before it would take effect. When he felt some relief, he would collapse from exhaustion from having worked so hard to breathe.

Our doctor in St. Louis helped us. He properly regulated the Theophyllin level and started him on a single shot weekly. Kirk improved some. Numerous asthma attacks still occurred. On the doctor's advice, we purchased a breathing machine to use at home and to eliminate some frantic trips to the hospital. (I found it extremely hard to remain calm on the surface when gripped with terror that the child may not survive this attack. (We never let Kirk know how frightened we were.)

Our St. Louis doctor stated that **in time** he might outgrow this asthma. **But when?** How many times could a child be held in the clutches of this agonizing struggle for breath? The doctor said when he can breathe no longer, he will pass out or lose consciousness: then, his muscles will relax, and he will resume breathing automatically. How can I be **sure**? The emotional strain of all this anxiety affected our whole family. My husband lost sleep, also. The commotion surrounding those night trips and the home attacks sometimes woke the other children. We were all losing sleep with the result that tensions were affecting the entire family. I believe that **Asthma** is a disease that afflicts the whole family whether or not more than one individual has it.

After each trip to St. Louis, the doctor would increase the amount of Theophyllin. Kirk was taking antihistamines and Alupent, in addition to the Theo daily. We were using the breathing machine not just occasionally but two, three, five or more times daily. Short-term doses of Prednisone were resumed. And antibiotics. For several months, Kirk did not sleep well at night.

Then, we learned about Dr. C. H. Robertson through an article in the *Evansville Courier & Press*. We read with interest of the story of Brandy Wilhite, an asthmatic child helped by Dr. Robertson and currently doing without medication. I consulted a doctor about this treatment (as outlined in the article), and he said it would be too risky to withdraw Kirk's medication. This doctor thought the diet might help (certainly couldn't hurt), but that diet could not cure him.

We laid the article aside, but from time to time I would pick it up and read it. Finally after much prayer and a plea for guidance, I picked up the telephone and called Dr. Robertson's office. My husband and I drove to Owensboro with some misgiving, but we were willing to try anything that might save the life of our son.

We talked to Kirk about Brandy Wilhite and told him that he had the same kind of breathing problems Kirk had and that Dr. Robertson had made him well. Kirk was eager to meet Dr. Robertson, and whatever fears he had about going to still another doctor were dispelled when Dr. Robertson picked him up and placed him on the table for examination. His friendly matter-of-fact approach won Kirk's confidence immediately. When he told him he wouldn't hurt him or anyone else—except the devil, they became good friends. Kirk listened attentively while he told him about the poisons in his body that must be removed—and that he must eat only *good* food.

Kirk's father and I listened too: When Dr. Robertson said "and no more medication" we were uneasy. But we had come this far (after much thought and prayer), and we determined to go whole-heartedly with Dr. Robertson's advice. As he talked, his advice sounded reasonable. All the months and months of medication had left their impact on Kirk's small body and had not made him well. Dr. Robertson's own faith freely expressed increased our confidence. As he explained to us the effect of chemicals in the body and how eating the right nutrients could help to eliminate Kirk's underlying problems, we began to think that perhaps God had guided us to the right source.

Kirk listened intently as Dr. Robertson explained that he was going to give him supplements—not drugs—to cure his body. He started him on seaweed, Veico, Vitamin C, and others. He convinced Kirk that fresh fruit and vegetables along with various nuts and seeds would help him develop a healthy body. He also succeeded in convincing him that sugar, in its refined state, was bad. Consequently, we have had no trouble with Kirk's remaining on his diet because Dr. Robertson took the time to explain to him the reasons for this treatment.

On our first day at Dr. Robertson's, the doctor gave Kirk several osteopathic treatments. He performed nasal surgery to open up Kirk's sinuses. He used a suction machine to remove mucous accumulations. Each time, he told Kirk what he was going to do and why. By evening Kirk had had no medicine all day. When he would start wheezing, Dr. Robertson would give him another treatment. We were amazed that he could breathe at all without the medicine. Usually, if he went an hour past his medication time he would be in trouble. The first night, he was wheezing and getting tight in his chest. He asked for a breathing treatment so he would not have "to go to the hospital and get a shot." My husband and I had begun to have misgivings. Everything Dr. Robertson said seemed so simple and contradictory to everything all the other doctors had said.

Dr. Robertson told Kirk he needed more exercise and that to expand his lungs he should run until he was exhausted. Before he had not exercised much because any labored breathing sometimes brought on an attack.

That first week was a long one. When we left Owensboro on Friday evening, we no longer doubted Dr. Robertson, and we knew we were on the right track. We continued to pray for strength and guidance in the care of this child and his brothers.

Kirk has been going to Dr. Robertson now for seven months. After the first week we spent at the clinic, we continued to go two or three times a week, then once a week, and now we are going once every two or three weeks because Kirk has improved so much.

The past six weeks he has not suffered an asthma attack. If he wheezes, we can handle it. A few extra glasses of honey and vinegar water and some vinegar packs will stop it.

Kirk is a different child. He looks great, and, he has grown in height. Our family life is different and wholesome. Our new knowledge of proper foods has benefited the entire family. We have learned to eat the right things.

Knowing the bewilderment and terror that can be a part of parenting such a child, I would like to be a beacon directing other parents to the satisfaction we have found through Dr. Robertson. To know that we can help our children combat and overcome this frightening ailment by simple and common sense nutrition is a gift from God.

Kirk has been a teacher to all of us—and especially to his peer group by relating the bad effects of sugar and junk foods. He is quick to point out to adults that certain things they eat are bad for them. Dr. Robertson has made a disciple of him. Kirk says maybe he will be a doctor. If so, I hope he will have the ability and compassion of the one who healed him.

Russelle Lear Boster
302 E. Douglas
Fairfield, Illinois 62837

> P.S. This summer Kirk has been taking swimming lessons. He rides his bike and jumps vigorously on the trampoline. He is full of energy and vitality. It has been a happy summer for him—and for us!

Mrs. Boster writes that Kirk became a disciple. Well, I do not know about that, but I do know he was an excellent patient, entering enthusiastically into treatments once he understood the reasons and implications of both

Asthma and Emphysema

treatments and diet recommendations. And Kirk wrote a "book" about his experience. If you wish to read Kirk's version of his odyssey, please turn to Appendices A and B entitled "The Allergy Story" and "The Allergy Kid."

Chapter IX

ARTHRITIS AND ARTHROSIS

Arthritis and/or arthrosis is evident in every living person whose diet consists of cooked foods. Remembering, then, that the body can only be as complete and sufficient as the nutrition entering that body, you could say that the body begins to degenerate as soon as it is born, if not before.

CAUSES AND SIGNS OF ARTHRITIS

Arthritis begins in the cell and is in every cell of the body as evidenced by the presence of toxins and the degeneration resulting from deficiency. As in any body disorder, toxins and deficiences cause the symptoms. The quality of every cell in the body determines an individual's health and health awareness.

Although most of us suffer from arthritis (or arthrosis) to some extent, we identify more advanced cases by swelling and inflammation of joints, occasionally even deformity, or by impairment of a part of the body because of pain occurring in varying degrees.

Most supposedly healthy people also will notice indications of arthritis after exercise—from the pain, soreness, and/or swelling which follow. Tissue used during exercise is being torn down constantly, rebuilt, and replaced. And the body performs this rebuilding, or attempt at rebuilding, through blood cells. Studies show that every cell in the body is renewed completely at least every seven years.

It is normal for toxins to develop from this tearing down of tissue and to accumulate in the exercised parts of the body, but lack of proper circulation and drainage allows these toxins to accumulate because they are not eliminated properly. Since it is more difficult for pathological tissue (abnormal tissue) to circulate and drain than for normal tissue to do so, the soreness following exercise would evidence arthritis, the process which includes repair. Thus, inflammation indicating arthritis derives from degenerating cells preventing proper elimination of accumulated toxins, as well as indicating the healing process.

CAUSES AND SIGNS OF ARTHROSIS

It is arthrosis we objectively see in deformed areas, in bone changes, in destruction of bone, cartilage, and soft tissue seen (on x-rays) as well as felt subjectively by the patient. Some arthrosis is visible in enlarged formations in and around joints.

In arthrosis, bone deteriorates, becomes rarefied (made rare, thin, porous, or less dense). As bone marrow and periosteum (the hard, outer covering of the bone) deteriorate and disintegrate, cartilage—the hard padding of the joint between bones—also may disappear. As a consequence, bones rub together, causing parts of them to wear off, disintegrate, or disappear.

Cartilage consists mostly of collagenous material. This collagen, a protein material similar to scar tissue, is a reinforcement nature creates to prevent destruction where two parts could rub together and cause wear. When this cartilage begins to disappear as it deteriorates, nature then causes swelling by rushing blood, lymph, and other body fluids to the area. This activity causes a barrier to build—a buffer—to prevent further damage from use while the area heals. Swelling and inflammation are natural conditions nature provides to correct a faulty condition, and will only remain as long as needed. Nature never ceases attempting to heal, to replace what has been lost or destroyed in the body.

Hard factual evidence of this ability was demonstrated to me in the case of Arnold Gerhardstein from Toledo, Ohio.

THE CASE OF ARNOLD GERHARDSTEIN

Some years ago, Arnold's mother phoned telling me about her two-year-old son. Neither of his hips had finished developing, and he lacked the ball and socket of the hip joints in the pelvis. When she brought Arnold Jr. to our clinic, he walked with a hobble and limped as if he had no hips.

As I began to work with the boy, I treated his body with osteopathic manipulation, working around the soft tissue of his hips and on his spinal and thigh muscles, attempting to create a condition in the area of the hip conducive to normal use—motion and function. The mother expertly cared for her boy, who stayed with us for five weeks, following the program we prescribed. During that period, we fed him a diet of fresh weeds from our own orchard and garden vegetables, mixed into salads. These leafy weeds consisted of dandelion, wild lettuce, plantain, narrow dock, sour dock, sour grass, sorrell, wild clover, blackberry leaves, tender young leaves of the sassafras tree, lamb's quarter and other wild grasses. As I recall, Arnold ate nothing cooked for those five weeks. At the end of that period, he had quit limping and continued to improve.

Rather than x-ray him at that time, the mother chose to wait and have it done at the clinic in Toledo, Ohio, where she had been told Arnold would never enjoy normal use of his hips. One year later, she called me to relay the results of x-rays just taken by her hometown doctor. I can still remember her excited words: "You won't believe this. The clinic says that this impossible thing that existed in Arnold's hips has changed entirely and he now has new hip balls and sockets."

Arthritis and Arthrosis

In 1982, about twenty years after seeing Arnold for the first time, I received a call from San Diego, California. The caller asked "Do you remember me, I'm Arnold Gerhardstein, Sr.?" I said "I certainly do, how's your little boy?" His reply warmed my heart: "You wouldn't believe him. Arnold Jr. is grown, he has a good body, and is a race car driver..."

I learned from this case as well as others never to believe that anything is impossible. The love and dedication of these parents had secured Arnold's future. They had moved to Mexico where they could obtain an abundance of fresh naturally-grown fruits and vegetables and, fortunately, found a home in the mountains with fresh pure air and a hot mineral spring not far from the house. Arnold was lucky to be able to begin his early years with good nutrition. I continually see, however, this healing process in all ages; early age is not a significant factor.

THE CASE OF LARRY HAMMOND

I remember a man past fifty, Larry Hammond, who had lost a hip, when his hip joint and the end of the femur and socket were destroyed by an airplane propeller. The man had been walking toward the door to board the plane. Thinking his passenger was already on board, the pilot started the propellers. Suddenly, the plane twisted and the propeller struck the man and tore up the upper end of his thigh. When he came to our clinic some years later, he limped terribly.

X-rays he brought along confirmed that the hip socket, the ball (the femur head), and the hip joint were destroyed. We began his treatments and placed him on a raw, natural diet. After several weeks of this treatment, resulting in great improvement, and after returning periodically for some time, we again x-rayed Larry. To his surprise, he had a new hip joint. The thigh had produced a ball and the socket had developed. The body's miraculous ability to correct or attempt to correct what is wrong never ends.

Symptoms merely warn us that something is amiss so that we may assist in rehabilitation.

TREATMENT: CLEANSING, DETOXIFICATION, DIET

Since arthritis and arthrosis result from degeneration, then treatment naturally would be to stop degeneration and begin regeneration. This process is done basically the same as mentioned throughout this book for most other disease conditions of the body.

First Step. The first step is to cleanse and detoxify the patient and to teach the person how to continue this process of keeping the system clean.

Second Step. The second step is to feed the patient proper foods to rejuvenate, rehabilitate, and reform the body successfully. We teach the patient to eat only fresh, poison-free, whole, natural foods—raw as much as possible—and grown on fertile soil. At the same time we explain that the

patient must eliminate toxic-forming foods and substances. The following items should be eliminated:
1. Chemically contaminated or polluted water;
2. Devitalized, degerminated, chemically treated, and synthetically enriched grain products. (For example, all refined cereals, breads, and pastries);
3. Unnecessary cooking of food;
4. Devitalized, sterilized, pasteurized, and ultra-pasteurized milk or milk products;
5. All refined sugars and hydrogenated fats and oils. (One of the worst habits for anyone, whether suffering from arthritis or not, is eating refined sugars. Laboratory test animals inevitably develop arthritis from eating refined sugars. And scientists, while analyzing synthetic glucose in the lab, discovered that sugar is a powerful decalcifier and magnet as it withdraws calcium into the bloodstream from the body tissue.)

Third Step. The third step is to encourage and assist the patient in exercise. Exercise is *most* necessary since it increases circulation, thereby increasing blood flow to affected areas, while aiding in elimination of toxins from those areas.

As long as a person lives, nature will *never* quit attempting to heal, repair, rebuild. Although some scar tissue will remain, some can be absorbed and eliminated by the body. Exercise should be applied according to the patient's condition, the areas affected, and with the patient's comfort in mind. The whole body should be exercised, for without it the body will atrophy (lose its function) and deteriorate. Bear in mind that the human brain and mind also atrophy and deteriorate if not exercised.

And a most definite part of Step Three is to ensure that all body parts are in structural order and normal position. This goal can be achieved in most cases by a physician trained in structural analysis, interpretation, and treatment.

Formerly, for these methods, the osteopathic physicians probably were the best trained, whereas today many osteopathic physicians have abandoned these methods and to some lesser degree, have relegated this approach to the chiropractor and professional therapest. I for one have not abandoned this valuable osteopathic approach; rather I have demonstrated successfully that the osteopathic approach is scientific and works.

Chapter X
CANCER, DETOXIFICATION, AND NUTRITION

Thirty years ago I shared a lecture platform at a Food and Farming Convention with Father Lyle Sheen, a cousin to the noted Bishop Sheen. In his address, he described cancer as a disease of *filth*. After forty-eight years of experience, I must still agree with him.

Through these years I have discovered that if we pursue a plan of detoxifying the body, removing it from environmental poisons as much as possible, feeding it fresh, pure, poison-free, organically grown food, and correcting the abnormal structure, most always any tumor in the body will cease to grow and will recede. Recently I examined two patients from Michigan and Pennsylvania who have had tumors shrink and absorbed eventually by their body after they completed their treatments.

Two years ago, I talked with a friend whose wife underwent a cancer operation involving her uterus. He explained to me that the doctor told them that because the cancer was localized in the uterus, which was removed, it could not invade again because it no longer had any connection with the blood stream. I asked my friend, "if it has not originally come from the blood stream, where did it originate?"

Not only in medical schools but also in elementary school health classes and high school home economics and biology classes, we are taught that certain foods build certain parts of our bodies and that this process occurs through our blood. If body tissue growth must come from food we eat, then at the same time any growth on this body tissue must also come from the same source. Even in the case of a tissue graft or organ transplant, the new part must still receive its food from the blood. So, logically, good blood can remove the same tumor that bad blood created.

We hear much disagreement about using laetril on cancer. Although I do not use it, evidence indicates that laetril does destroy tumor cells without toxic effect on the body. Regardless of what destroys the tumor, however, it is all the more necessary to detoxify the body of all causative agents which first produced the tumor.

I cannot emphasize enough the notion that the body, with its law of the blood (a natural law), never does anything wrong. Daily, I am aware constantly of the power of blood to move the body toward health.

Any natural food store carries scores of books by or about people who have conquered cancer by nutritional means. Two excellent books by Robert Stickle, *Cancer: One Man's Fight to Control Malignancy* and *A Rational Concept of Cancer*, describe how Stickle overcame a severe melanoma and emphasize that the patient must first desire to get well, believe he can, and be determined to do so. He also stresses that the patient accept *no* treatment that destroys tissue unless such treatment does not affect any other part of the body.

When a person destroys a part of the body by radiation or some other such means, that person sins against God. The marriage declaration "What (not just who) God has joined together, let no man put asunder" also applies to a person's body. We cannot create a state of health by killing or eliminating a necessary part.

Today's "horror of cancer" lies not in cancer itself but in our commonly practiced methods for treatment of cancer. I well remember my own shock and disbelief when told many years ago that I probably had cancer in an internal organ. Luckily for me, this incident happened about the same time I had begun to learn and to apply principles of natural living. Now, forty years later, I am in excellent health, and for years have had no indication of cancer—and, as I recall, worried little about ever having it.

In those early years of learning and practicing the principles of natural healing, I was influenced by books and people's experiences. I remember, for example, a lady who came to the clinic with this story: "One of your patients asked me to come and show you a hopeless cancer victim who became well after giving up. Someone told me I could cure myself of cancer with fresh, organically-grown juices, which I did with the use of a vegetable press." I can still see the lady as she spoke: she spoke with great vitality, and her face was filled with healthy color and rosy cheeks. After thirty years, I hear she is still alive and healthy.

Cancer is a condition created by the presence of poison or toxins in the blood. The tumor is only the effect. The tumor demonstrates causally the body's vitality or ability to remove poison from the body and to channel it to one spot or spots. The tumor acts as the dump or waste basket for the poison. Technically and scientifically, when a person has cancer, it indicates that the blood is overloaded with toxins. But society is taught to believe that cancer or a cancerous tumor is localized, and when that part is removed or destroyed, the cancer is gone. I find it difficult to believe that doctors truly believe this, especially when I hear so many of them say to me: "I know radiation and chemotherapy are wrong, and I'd never use it on myself, but I don't know any alternatives."

I am convinced that cancer always begins in the blood. It is more prevalent today, in our lifetime, because there are more poisons than there ever have been. Our air and water are polluted; our food is adulterated, fumigated, and poisoned by pesticides. The body was designed with the facility to handle and eliminate poisons up to a certain limit, but we are reaching this limit. Therefore, it is important to obtain maximum nutrition from our food intake and to attain maximum functioning from our eliminatory organs, which we can only do if we clean the blood by cleaning the sewer. Cancer is no big complex mystery; it is, simply, a disease of filth.

Cancer, Detoxification & Nutrition

I have watched both types of leukemia, myelogenous (bone marrow) and lymphatic (of the lymph system), respond well to good nutrition and detoxification, because both originate as a result of improper nutrition and toxins which destroy the blood-forming organs.

We must stop searching for one single savior in cancer treatment and attack the cause—degeneration of the total body resulting from many causes. Daily we hear of new findings of cancer-producing agents. People say to me, "What can I eat; everything produces cancer?" Well, we can eat a large variety of health-inducing foods. Certain facts will help in choosing a diet, free from cancer-producing foods. We do know that cancerous growths require sugar to grow: also, tests prove that rancid (decomposing) oils and fats are dangerous. An eastern university in this country discovered that rancid oils fed to test animals caused cancer to develop in one hundred percent of tested animals. Apparently, rancid oil decreases oxygenation (use of oxygen), decreasing the function of every cell. Because of the chemical nature (hydrogenation), the blood content becomes heavy, and the body cannot transport it well. The thickened blood acts as a drag in a water pipe that holds back or impedes flow. Thus, the body experiences a difficult time trying to eliminate the effects of the rancid oil through the liver, kidneys, bowel, and skin.

Rancid oils can come from hydrogenated oils and fats and from old or unrefrigerated oils, fats, nuts, and grains. Although hydrogenation supposedly prevents rancidity, some *does* occur because oil will oxidize—hydrogenation changes the nature of the oil so it cannot be digested or absorbed properly. Anytime a fresh grain is ground into flour, refined or unrefined, oils in this grain will oxidize and become rancid within a short time if not refrigerated. A good test to prove this process at home is to grind fresh whole wheat into flour and leave it exposed a few days to the elements. Then bake it into bread and eat it. Soon after, you should notice a lot of mucous discharge. Mucous, nature's method of eliminating toxins, is the vehicle by which your system frees itself of decomposing spoiled oil from the grain.

Any food known to cause cancer in test animals also can do the same for you. But one food will not necessarily cause cancer anymore than one miracle drug will heal it. I remember this statement from a teacher's remark that also applies to cancer: "All disease is due to substances the body needs and is not getting and to the presence of substances which the body contains and does not need."

We do not have to live in fear of cancer when we understand its cause.

Chapter XI

OUR CARDIO-VASCULAR SYSTEM

More than forty million men, women, and children in America have something wrong with their hearts or blood vessels. Each year, nearly one million die from cardiovascular diseases, mostly heart attacks and strokes. Dollar costs for medical services and losses in earnings and production are estimated at more than forty billion dollars yearly.

THE HEART'S TASK

Every day, the heart—much of it a muscle and hardly bigger than a clenched fist—pumps five to six quarts of blood through the 60,000 mile network of arteries, veins, and capillaries comprising the body's circulatory system to nourish trillions of body cells. The heart beats 100,000 times a day, pumping 2,500 - 5,000 gallons of blood. In a life-time, it will beat two and a half billion times and pump 100 million gallons of blood. Our arteries also pump as the heart does, contracting and relaxing the same as the heart, pumping and releasing.

HEART DAMAGE

When the normal blood flow from the heart to the body is impeded or when the blood supply that nourishes the heart itself is blocked, the heart can break down. The result is some form of "Heart Disease," or "Cardiovascular Disease" (*Cardio* meaning heart and *vascular* meaning blood vessels).

The heart cannot work without blood, which causes it to contract and keeps it nourished. When the blood supply shuts off, it cripples the heart. Not only the heart, but also all body parts must be nourished by blood. To impede or slow down normal circulation is to impede the performance of each body part. For the blood to reach the parts it must nourish, there must be a pressure adequate to force it there, and there must be proper functioning of the heart and valves. If a body part does not receive blood, it will cease to function. Any body part—heart, colon, or skin—will begin to atrophy if it receives inadequate nourishment from blood quality or quantity.

Heart diseases usually are named according to the part of the heart damaged. Subjective symptoms of heart problems might be abnormal flutter or irregular heart beat, a racing heart, one that skips beats or beats too slowly. Objective symptoms might be a swelling ankle caused by failure of the heart to keep circulation moving or by uneven heart-beat when heard with a stethescope.

Symptoms of a heart attack could be a mild or severe pain in the chest and/or even abdomen and/or difficulty in breathing. This pain is the body indicating that something is out of business.

A heart attack is caused most often when an artery closes, preventing blood supply to a part of the heart. The extent of the attack will depend on the extent of damage to the heart muscle when the blood supply was shut off and did not reach the muscle, and on how large an area of the muscle has been eliminated.

A heart attack can be caused by an embolism—a particle breaking loose somewhere in the body and ending up, more or less, in an end artery (an artery with no other way out). When the embolism, or particle, plugs up the little artery, it shuts off the blood supply to an area, leaving it without much blood which then causes an infarct - an area with scar tissue forming because of lack of blood supply. This scar tissue forms as nature reinforces the muscle which has had the blood supply eliminated.

Heart damage is caused by deficiency of the elements, plus the presence of toxins. As arteries degenerate, muscles lose their tone and the quality of the heart valves deteriorate. The weak and lazy valve prolapses (falls into its own space), and does not remain closed when it should.

Just as disintegrating teeth reflect deterioration proceeding in the body, varicose veins and hemorrhoids show this deterioration through collapsing blood vessels. As construction of the artery or vein wall disintegrates, the wall first will dilate, then thin out and balloon, resulting in the varicose vein, hemorrhoid or aneurysm if an artery.

Most heart and valve replacement-type surgery results from this deterioration and disintegration. Since all these parts—pericardium, myocardium, endocardium, and muscles—will deteriorate together, replacing only one part is no comprehensive solution.

In addition, a problem involving imperfect valves can result from the mother's deficiencies. A defect in construction of or damage to some of the heart valves—the valves separating the chambers of the heart—may be caused before birth or in early infancy. Toxins, furthermore, will prevent the valve from staying matured or developed, and allow it to disintegrate. A properly working valve is most necessary to hold back the blood pressure so that the heart can contract. This pressure is needed to force the blood to all parts of the body so they may be nourished.

UNDERLYING CAUSES OF HEART DAMAGE

ARTERIOSCLEROSIS

The major underlying cause of heart disease, stroke, and related disorders is arteriosclerosis or "hardening of the arteries." This degenerative disease can narrow or block, in time, arteries leading into the heart, brain, and other parts of the body as the artery wall hardens.

Our Cardio-Vascular System

Arteriosclerosis is a necessary pathological phenomenon. When the wall of the artery deteriorates from lack of sufficient nutrition, nature must reinforce it or it would otherwise burst. The deteriorating wall is rebuilt or reinforced with a fibrous tissue or a collagen-type material, which causes the arterial wall to become thicker than normal, or to calcify.

ATHEROSCLEROSIS

Accompanying arteriosclerosis will usually be atherosclerosis, a coating of the inside of the artery and subsequent obstruction of the artery by stopping it up. Atherosclerosis is a disease characterized by fatty degeneration of the inner coat of the arteries. Plaque accumulates on the artery's inner wall. As materials such as cholesterol and other fatty substances constantly circulating in the bloodstream push their way beneath injured arterial cells, they form deposits called plaques. As plaques build up, arterial walls roughen and begin to narrow as do the lumen or spaces, making it difficult for blood to pass through.

Dr. Richard Passwater, author of *Super Nutrition for Healthy Hearts*, explains that the plaque continues to grow because the cholesterol within the fibrous plaque attracts calcium from the bloodstream. This process complicates matters because the calcium not only adds a certain rigidity to the plaque but also attracts additional material from the bloodstream including more cholesterol, triglycerides, and other elements. As this attraction between calcium and cholesterol continues, the plaque grows in size, layer by layer.

I do not suggest, however, that cholesterol causes atherosclerosis. According to *Nutrition News*, "For many years physicians and scientists supported the theory that the cholesterol deposits accumulating in the arteries were caused by too much cholesterol in the diet. Electron microscope techniques, however, show that cholesterol appears only after the lesions, injuries to arterial walls, have formed. Also, studies show that cholesterol produced by the arterial cells facilitate the flow of the bloodstream."

Natural fats should not contribute to hardening of arteries or a fat buildup within the artery if these oils are not contaminated or perverted (as in the case of hydrogenation). Hydrogenation refers to the process of changing the nature of oil to prevent its spoilage. Hydrogenation perverts fats so the body cannot break down and digest these fats. Therefore, they partly become foreign bodies—toxins—the body must eliminate. Natural fats and oils will be digested properly by the stomach, and by secretions of the liver, pancreas, and small intestine. Eskimos and Chinese, living on high-fat diets, never suffered from hardening of arteries until they began to eat highly-processed, civilized foods.

HIGH BLOOD PRESSURE

As arteries narrow, the heart must work harder to circulate the blood, resulting in high blood pressure. Normal blood pressure is a natural phenomenon and is necessary to supply blood to every organ. Normal blood pressure is the force exerted by the blood against the arterial walls as your heart pumps blood through the arteries. Normally, each time the heart pumps (about sixty to seventy times a minute), it pushes blood out into the arteries (the tubes that carry blood from the heart to the lungs, kidneys, brain, and other vital organs). The blood then returns to the heart through the veins.

Uncontrolled high blood pressure, also called hypertension, leads to atherosclerosis by damaging the normally smooth lining of the arteries, which then allows the plaque accumulation. This accumulation can lead to blockage of an artery supplying blood to the heart—resulting in a heart attack, or it can lead to blockage of an artery leading to the brain—producing a stroke.

High blood pressure affects some forty to sixty million Americans and can be present for years without exhibiting visible symptoms. It is the leading secondary cause of strokes and a major factor in heart attacks and kidney failure.

Two other contributing factors to high blood pressure are increased viscosity (thickening) of the blood, and ptosis, (falling or dropping of abdominal organs). Ptosis will cause an added strain and embarrassment on circulation through the kidneys and adrenal bodies, as the abdominal organs pull downward on the kidneys. Dropped organs also may act as a wedge in the pelvis and shut off some circulation to the legs, causing the body to raise the blood pressure to force the blood through this dam.

Recently a friend told me of a medical journal article mentioning the change in viscosity of blood as one cause of high blood pressure. This blood viscosity, plus areas in the body where the arterial bed is already tight, accounts for ninety-five percent of all high blood pressure in America.

These tight and narrowed vessels, which obstruct normal arterial flow, essentially result from mineral deficiencies occurring during a long period of time, perhaps in many cases having begun in the nutrition of the mother and even earlier generations. This condition would be familial, not hereditary as we are led to believe. As mentioned elsewhere, hereditary factors remain important only insofar as bad dietary habits are carried from generation to generation. This is why I believe that no disease manifestation is carried by genes.

Blood viscosity is evident when the blood is toward the alkaline side. The more alkaline something becomes, the thicker it becomes. As blood becomes more relatively alkaline, it becomes thicker, automatically demanding a higher pressure to move it through the finer capillaries to assure that all parts of the body receive adequate amounts of blood.

Alkalosis can be caused by eating predominantly alkaline-forming foods such as cooked foods and highly alkaline foods, and by drinking water with a high lime content. Nearly all foods are alkaline-forming except prunes, plums, honey, vinegar, apples, cranberries, seaweed, and distilled water. Leafy green vegetables, when eaten raw, also would be safe since nature would control their alkalinity through the skin, kidneys, and lungs. Certain types of acid foods help prevent deposits in the veins, joints, gall bladder, and kidneys without causing too much alkalinity. As examples, I prefer natural apple cider vinegar, good wine vinegars, grape juice (tartaric acid) and grapefruit juice from the pulp (citric acid). Dr. Jarvis' book (mentioned earlier) is an excellent source on learning about alkalosis of the blood. Thus, correcting one's diet can serve as the most immediate means to correct a heart problem. Arteriosclerosis and atherosclerosis naturally require some time to correct. We do know that vitamin C and the bio-flavanoids will help to dissolve cholesterol, and Mg and B6 will help to dissolve plaques in blood vessels.

OUR TREATMENT FOR HEART DAMAGE AND DISEASE

In a recent women's magazine article, a physician wrote on high blood pressure. The first third of the article explained hypertension, the second dealt with statistics, and the final third described in detail drugs to treat and control this disease. He also mentioned the relationship to salt, smoking, and drinking habits. At the beginning of this final third of his article, he stated that "the major underlying cause of heart disease, stroke, and related disorders is arteriosclerosis—a degenerative disease." Why did he not even indicate anywhere in the entire article that since the case was *de*generative, the cure must be *re*generative?

From my own practice, I know that regeneration can be achieved, as it must be achieved to keep arteries clear and the blood slippery through proper diet, detoxification, exercise, and any necessary structural correction. If you want a healthy heart, you must eliminate refined foods, chemically-deranged water, and approach a ninety-percent raw diet. Liberally use apple cider vinegar and pure honey, which can be used in the drink "huniger" and applied directly on your food. Clean fresh air with adequate exercise is also necessary, along with a positive attitude.

When a person comes to our clinic suffering from a heart attack, we first ease the patient with an osteopathic treatment to relieve the fibrosis or the spasm in the area of the spine that controls the blood supply to the heart. The pain usually can be stopped or relieved by relaxing the spinal nerve center to the heart. Next, we clean the patient out, as we attempt to eliminate a part of the cause. Detoxifying, cleaning the bowel and freeing the body of toxins, helps the body operate with less impairment. Then we proceed with a diet of vegetable juices, such as carrot, parsley, beet, cabbage, and wheat grass. Celery is especially good because of its content of silica which increases the strength of the wall of the cell. This program of detoxification and rebuilding the blood and body through proper nutrition is continued for as long as needed. The diet becomes the person's lifestyle which enables him to lead a long, healthy life, free from the fear that someday he will be senile, useless, and unable to enjoy the pleasures of children, grandchildren, and great-grandchildren.

Chapter XII

FEMALE PROBLEMS

HYSTERECTOMIES

I believe, along with many of my associates, that hysterectomies frequently are unnecessary. In most cases, when the patient's total condition is analyzed, physicians will discover the uterus is out of place, tilted, crowded, and held out of place by adhesions. These conditions usually result from faulty intestinal position. Pressure from the fallen bowel—a result of weak ligaments caused by a low state of nutrition—will result invariably in this frequency of faulty uterine positioning. Since all abdominal organs are connected (more or less), when one falls or slips out of position, all the others automatically will be pulled down or affected. If these defective, structural problems are corrected and necessary changes in the diet implemented to prevent recurrence (plus proper attention to normal elimination), most hysterectomies could be and should be avoided. *Hysterectomy should only be the final procedure if conservative measures fail.*

CRAMPS AND MENSTRUAL PAIN

During the menstrual period, cramps result most often from obstruction of the cervix and faulty positioning of the uterus. Frequently, they also can result from twisted Fallopian tubes caused by the uterus's abnormal position. Many of these abnormal positions generally are correctable manually, or through application of a uterine spoon by a physician, in his office, without surgical cutting. This spoon is an instrument invented by Dr. Andrew Taylor Still in the 1800's after the Civil War to correct a faulty uterine position not correctable by hand.

Ovarian pain, or pain or discomfort near the ovaries, can result from the tubes as they are twisted by uterine misplacement resulting from bowel ptosis and loss of ligamentous tone from malnutrition.

This same low state of nutrition, or malnutrition, also can cause fibrosis to develop within ligaments holding organs in place. Fibrous tissue will shorten as scar tissue does; likewise, as these ligaments age, they will shorten. This shortening of ligaments will pull on the uterus and inevitably result in pain around the ovaries. The fibrotic ligaments will remain so, unless stretched and corrected either manually or through use of a uterine spoon, which can be done in a doctor's office over a period of time. This procedure is executed by freeing the twisted tubes from their bondage by repositioning the uterus and loosening the adhesions adjacent to the reproductive organs, and by repositioning the abdominal organs (mainly the bowel — the large and small intestines).

Most menstrual pain derives from obstruction in the uterine cervix. Most often, immediate causes include deformity of the cervical canal and/or overgrowth of the canal wall, which narrows the passage. This problem allows the body of the uterus to hold the menstruum, while preventing the proper opening during contraction of the uterine muscle as it attempts to force the emptying of the flow. This observation can be verified easily by replacing the faulty uterine position and dilating the cervix instrumentally by a competent physician who understands the cause.

IRREGULARITY

Besides being caused by a low fiber diet, as we are all aware of today, bowel irregularity also can be caused by defective positioning of the female and/or abdominal organs, from endocrine disorders, or from partial obstruction of the cervical canal—the opening of the uterus. All these conditions result from a low state of nutrition of the patient (plus errors in nutrition by his ancestors). This judgment does not indicate that the problem itself is hereditary, but that the deficiency causing the problem is *familial* in the diet and living habits.

Bladder symptoms frequently occur in uterine malpositions because of bladder distortion by the uterus and colon. In hysterectomies, adhesions resulting from surgery can cause hazardous effects to the bladder or urethra.

SPOTTING AND HEMORRHAGING

Spotting is most often caused by an obstructed, cervical canal. It also can be caused by swelling of the womb from congestion, by bleeding tumors in the cervix or the womb's interior, or by womb erosions or ulcers.

Hemorrhaging in female organs also can result from varicose veins in the uterus. To shrink these veins naturally, the uterus can be treated with packs soaked in natural apple cider vinegar. Many doctors apply this vinegar pack remedy today to internal swelling and bleeding.

These conditions are not only amenable to this swelling reduction treatment, but also are nearly always amenable to conservative treatment. I am convinced that the safest approach to cancer of these organs is this conservative treatment, and not radical removal.

THE CASE OF LOLITA BOGDAN

Daily, in using the conservative treatment, I see cases similar to Lolita Bogdan, who began her menopause at thirty-seven. At the beginning, her

Female Problems

periods were irregular with flooding on the first and second days. A few months later, she agreed to a currettage, a scraping of the interior of the uterus (although her doctor recommended a complete hysterectomy). After this scraping, and during each period for the next ten months, Lolita experienced cramping and hemorrhaging with gigantic clots. The following four months, the bleeding began every two weeks. Naturally, her iron count dropped low. Fearing that one more period could cause her to bleed to death, and on the advice of friends, Lolita came to our clinic. We discovered her uterus to be thick, swollen, and spongy; and we observed a high estrogen count, close to cancerous.

For the next three weeks, Lolita's treatment consisted of daily treatments of osteopathic manipulation and structural correction of her uterine position. Her diet and water were changed, and vitamin and mineral supplements were added. After the first day, we observed a slight improvement, and by the end of three weeks, her hemorrhaging had ceased, the swelling had gone down, and her uterus looked much like a healthy organ. Before long, her periods were normal, with scant clotting or cramps. Now, we see Lolita only periodically for maintenance and some structural help through her menopause.

HEADACHES ASSOCIATED WITH CONSTIPATION AND/OR DIARRHEA

The actual causative location of most headaches is primarily in the upper rectal area and the adjacent segment of colon—the sigmoid and/or iliac pelvic colon. The structural problem in this area invariably results from degeneration of the bowel from eating devitalized food. As organs degenerate, the following happens: varicose veins form within the anatomical parts, the bowel wall thins, the muscle wall degenerates and becomes less active, and fibrosis—nature's plan to reinforce to compensate for weakness—begins.

All of these conditions will respond to correct nutrition and conservative treatment, involving structural correction of the positioning of the involved organs. I have never seen a case of migraine headaches which did not respond to this procedure. In most migraine headache cases, there also exists pressure from the ptosed abdominal organs on the reproductive organs and the colon's pelvic parts.

TUMORS OF UTERUS OR OVARIES

The most common tumors of these organs is the humble fibroid of the uterus (which may grow as large as a grapefruit) and the fibroid-like tumor of the ovaries, usually smaller. Cysts of the ovaries would be the next most common.

We know we can produce cysts in laboratory animals through a diet of refined flour, pasteurized milk, cooked meat, and refined sugars. I have observed the same result in human beings. It follows, therefore, to correct the described condition, that all offending agents be eliminated, the body detoxified, and proper correction be completed on all organs involved. The abdominal organs always need to be replaced to proper position if at all possible—manually, by degravitization, or by proper ptosis support.

Fibroids, other growths, and cysts invariably and without exception will begin to disappear as the diet is corrected and structural corrections are completed. They will be annihilated, destroyed, and/or absorbed and eliminated by the lymph and ultimately by the blood. Depending on the size of the growth and the patient's cooperation, this procedure can require months, weeks, or only a few days. I remind my patients that they must not expect what took years to develop to disappear overnight. For with time, decomposition of the abnormal growth can be cared for by autolytic enzymes and ferments provided by nature for restoration to the normal body blueprint.

STERILITY

Much, perhaps most, sterility today—based on research performed on test animals—is thought to result from the following:

1. Devitalized, degerminated, overheated cereal grain products;
2. Pasteurized milk and milk products; and
3. Cooked meat, particularly meat from animals fed synthetics, hormones, and antibiotics.

If true with test animals, it follows that most likely the same result—given the same diet—is inevitable in human beings.

As you may have discovered by now in the preceding paragraphs, our treatment reverses or removes the cause. The diet causing the problem must be corrected, and the structural problems also must be corrected.

Besides beginning a wholesome, fresh, natural, poison-free, nutritious diet (aided by thorough chewing), it is imperative, regardless of the condition, that the patient eliminate the following: chemically-treated water, hydrogenated fats, all milk products, refined and/or enriched flours and cereals, refined sugars, tobacco, strong drugs, and carbonated and sugared drinks.

The restorative process is fantastic in the way organs will respond to repositioning when no longer starved for mineral food. The body never ceases to try to heal or recover.

The conservative structural correction must be done by the physician. To reposition the uterus, he will need to dilate and to restructure the cervix and cervical canal either manually or with the uterine spoon. To correct the ptosed or dropped bowel, he may follow several practices. We use the following:

Female Problems

1. Manipulating the abdominal content, directing it upward or at least toward normal position;
2. Degravitizing the body so gravity will help correct the ptosis;
3. Having the patient wear a ptosis support which helps lift the abdominal content, for a period of time (usually rather consistently for two years);
4. Instrumentally with a sigmoidoscope correcting the rectal and/or sigmoid deformity and adhesions through or within the rectum and into the sigmoid colon. (Additional help will be attained with the skilled use of the colonoscope.);
5. Using herbal laxatives, and natural bulk to improve bowel tone, elimination, and mobility;
6. Teaching the patient to rejuvenate the intestinal flora by taking acidophilus orally, and by acidophilus implant, until the normal flora is reestablished.

Also, we urge patients to recognize and use wild garden weeds in raw salads—most effective in reculturing the colon's normal flora population. A word of caution, it is an established fact that use of antibiotics is fatal to normal intestinal flora, which is attested to by the label on most, if not all, antibiotic products.

CONCLUSION

For too long, medical reasoning depended upon theory principally pragmatic and to much lesser extent on laws of science (which are infallible). If, however, an idea is absolutely scientific ever, it is always scientific. The point simply is that if medicine is to exist in any form it must be absolutely scientific.

Today, physicians are challenged on all fronts: Do physicians teach and practice these absolute laws of science (God's irrefutable laws) or do physicians still follow pagan ideas handed down for more than two thousand years?

Two dominant assertions have controlled medical practice:

1) Dedication of all medical practitioners to the first portion of the Hippocratic Oath which in effect is a pledge to heathen gods and goddesses, and

2) A later part—not law—which says Medicine and *religion* must remain separate.

Both of these statements violate all Judeo-Christian principles and beliefs of some other religions.

Neither of these assertions deserves respect among medical practitioners in any age of civilization even partly characterized as respecting and employing scientific methods.

If the reader has not gathered from the preceding chapters the following, I hereby restate two fundamentals:

1) Laws of science absolutely govern the state of health in your body.

2) Also, laws of science absolutely govern all processes of the disease state. We do not find mysterious the disease process. I beg you to study your body and to learn how to ensure it never does anything wrong.

If I may, let me refresh and reiterate the cardinal points I hope you will apply:

1) Provide your body with fresh, poison-free food (whole and mostly raw);

2) Learn to cleanse your body inside and out and to keep it clean;

3) *Fix* (or employ someone who knows how to) your body machine. Remember, your body must be mechanically in order, just as your car's parts must be structurally in order.

I challenge you, dear reader, to practice these principles. If you do, you will enjoy a more abundant life.

GLOSSARY

Alkalosis - Abnormally high relative alkalinity of body tissues and fluids.

Allergy - Hypersensitivity to a specific substance or condition which in similar amounts is harmless to most people; manifests itself in a physiological disorder. An exaggerated or abnormal reaction to substances, situations, or physical states harmless to most people. A normal protective mechanism.

Antrum - A cavity; especially either of a pair of sinuses in the upper jaw (Maxilla).

Arteriosclerosis - Abnormal thickening and hardening of artery walls (especially of the intima).

Arthritis - Inflammation of a joint or joints and/or contiguous tissue.

Arthrosis - Atrophic degenerative and regenerative processes affecting a joint: existing bony change in joint or bone indicating nature's healing process.

Atheroma - A disease characterized by fatty degeneration of the inner-coat of the arteries, resulting in collection of plaques on and in the arterial wall, or in a breaking down of the intima—leading to an atheromatous ulcer.

Atherosclerosis - Artery disease characterized by patchy nodular thickenings of artery inner walls, especially at branch points.

Bacteria - Typically one-celled microorganisms which have no chlorophyll, multiply by simple division, and visible only with a microscope (same as flora and/or germs).

Cause - Anything producing an effect or result. A reason.

Colon - That part of the large intestine extending from the cecum to the rectum; normal length approximately five feet long; in today's living American adult, it extends about thirteen feet long.

Contaminate - To defile. To make impure, infected, corrupt, radioactive, etc. by contact with or addition of something; pollute; defile; sully, taint.

Detoxify - To remove a poison or a poisonous effect from the body or body part.

Disease - Generally, any deviation of the body from its normal or healthy state; a particular disorder with a specific cause and characteristic symptoms; a particular destructive process in an organ or organism, with a specific cause and characteristic symptoms; actually, the process of becoming well.

Drug - Any substance used as a medicine or as an ingredient in a medicine.

Ethmoid - Designating or of the perforated bone or bones forming part of the septum and walls of the nasal cavity; the olfactory nerves pass through the perforations.

Etiology - Assignment of a cause, the original science of causes or origins of disease; causes of a specific disease.

Fibrosis - Abnormal increase in the amount of fibrous connective tissue in an organ, part, or tissue.

Germ - The rudimentary form from which a new organism develops; seed, bud, etc.; that from which something can develop or grow; origin; basis; any microscopic organism, esp. one of the bacteria that plays a role in the body's recovery process.

Health - Physical and mental well-being; freedom from disease, pain, or defect; an optimum state of symptom-free living.

Hemorrhoid - Painful swelling of a vein in the region of the anus, often with bleeding.

Huniger - A Vermont folk medicine made by mixing one teaspoonful each of honey and apple cider vinegar and one eight-ounce glass of water.

Ill - Not healthy, normal, or well; having a disease; sick; indisposed.

Illness - The condition of being ill, or in poor health; sickness; disease; any deviation from optimal health.

Immunity - Resistance to or protection against a specified disease; power to resist infection, especially as a result of antibody formation.

Intestine - The tubular portion of the alimentary canal from the pyloric end of the stomach to the anus; the bowels. In man, the intestine is five or six times the length of the body and forms numerous convolutions in the abdominal cavity, being attached and supplied with blood and lymph vessels and nerves by the mesentery. Its walls, which contain numerous glands, consist of an internal mucous membrane, a submucosa, a muscular coat of two layers (the inner with circular, the outer with longitudinal fibres), and in most parts an external serous coat. Its muscles are nonstriated and perform peristaltic movements. The first four-fifths of the intestine constitutes the small intestine, comprising the duodenum, jejunum, and ileum; the remaining fifth, the large intestine, comprising the cecum, colon, and rectum and distinguished by its larger diameter, sacculated form, and by the absence of certain structures (villus, valvulae, conniventes) present in the small intestine. Besides serving to carry off waste matter, the intestine, especially the first part of it, is the seat of the completion of digestion on and (by means of the blood vessels and lacteals in its walls) of the absorption of nourishment. (By permission. From Webster's *New International Dictionary*, copyright 1927.)

Terms for Glossary

Intima - The tunica intima, or inner coat of a blood-vessel.

Medicine - The science and art of diagnosing, treating, curing, and preventing disease, relieving pain, and improving and preserving health.

Mesentery - A supporting membrane or membranes enfolding some internal organ and attaching it either to the body wall or to another organ; especially a double thickness of the peritoneum enfolding most of the small intestine and attaching it to the spinal wall of the abdominal cavity; tissue designed to carry nerve, blood, and lymph to and from abdominal and pelvic organs.

Plaques - Mounds of lipid material mixed with smooth muscle cells and calcium, which lodge in artery walls.

Pollute - To make unclean, impure, or corrupt; defile, contaminate; dirty.

Potion - A drink or liquid dose, as of medicine, or a supposedly magic substance.

Ptosis - A prolapse, or falling of some organ or organs.

Pylorus - Pyloric orifice; the aperture between the stomach and small intestine (duodenum).

Resistance - Ability of an organism to ward off disease; the act of resisting, opposing, withstanding, etc.; the power or capacity to resist.

Science - Systematized knowledge derived from observation, study, and experimentation conducted to determine the nature or principles of the subject studied, actual meaning never changing (infallible truth).

Serum - Any watery animal fluid; the thin watery part of a plant fluid.

Sigmoid Flexure - The final curving part of the colon, ending in the rectum; normally six to ten inches in a healthy bowel.

Sphenoid - Designating or of the wedge-shaped compound bone at the base of the skull, wedge-shaped; the sphenoid bone, containing one of the larger sinuses.

Stenosis - An abnormal narrowing, often with roughness, of any canal or passage in the body.

Stricture - A limiting or restricting condition; restriction; partial closure.

Superstition - Any belief or attitude, based on fear or ignorance, inconsistent with known laws of science or with that generally considered in the particular society as true and rational.

Telescoping - Having parts that slide one inside another, or are forced one into another.

Turgescent - To swell, becoming turgid or swollen; swelling; more discolored than normal (ordinarily bluish-red).

Turgid - Swollen; distended.

Vaccine - Any preparation of killed microorganisms, living weakened organisms, etc. introduced into the body theoretically and supposedly to produce immunity to a specific disease by causing formation of antibodies.

Varicose - Abnormally and irregularly swollen or dilated.

Virus - Any of a group of ultramicroscopic or submicroscopic infective agents theoretically causing various diseases in animals, as measles, mumps, etc., or in plants, as mosaic diseases; viruses are capable of multiplying only. in connection with living cells and are regarded both as living organisms and as complex proteins sometimes involving nucleic acid, enzymes, etc.

Viscosity - Quality or state of being viscous. The resistance offered by a fluid to the relative motion of its particles; internal friction.

Viscous - Adhesive or sticky, and having a ropy or glutinous consistency.

Volvulus - A twisting or displacement of intestine, resulting in intestinal obstruction; also looping or convoluting.

Appendix A
The Allergy Story by the Allergy Kid

The Allergy Story
by the
Allergy Kid

KIRK BOSTER

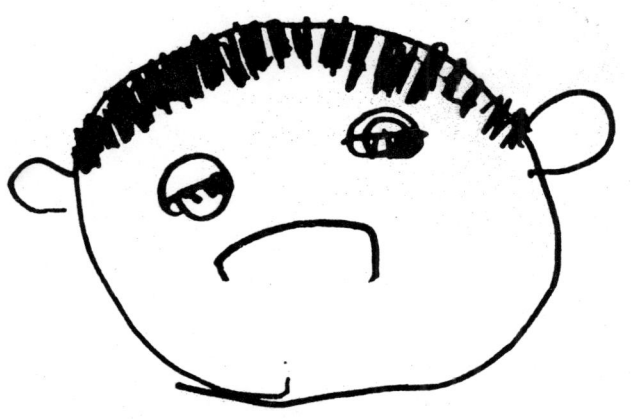

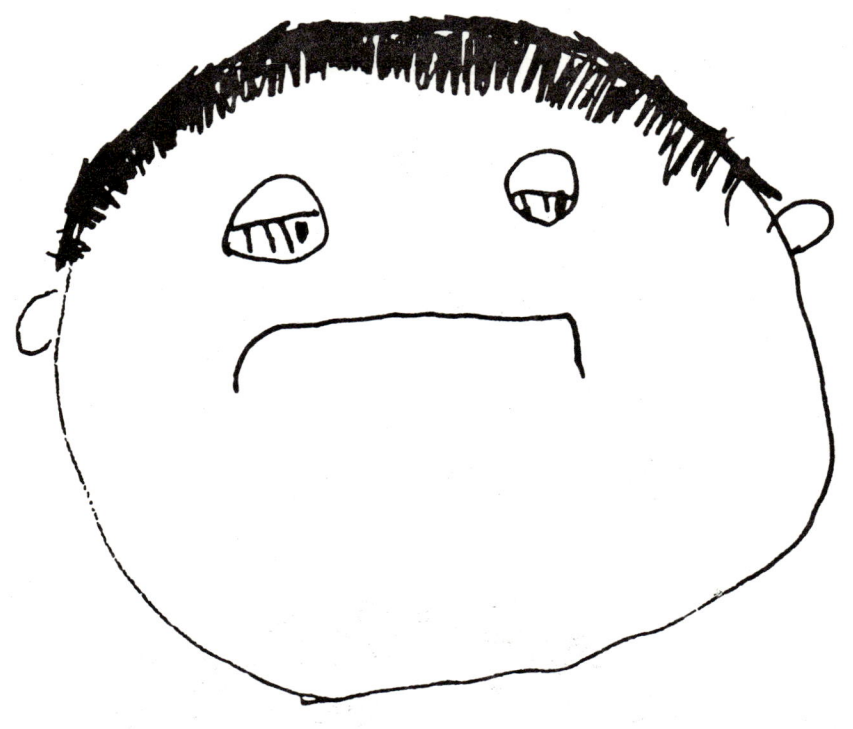

Sometimes I can't sleep very good because sometimes I get wheezy. My head goes up and down. My eyes get blurry. My tongue feels good but my gums feel bad. I get my Dad up and tell him I don't feel good.

Appendix A

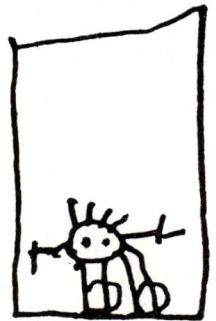 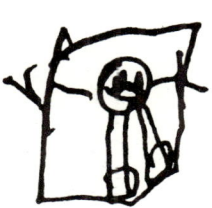

He piggy-backs to me to the kitchen and gives me pills. I go back to bed but I can't sleep so I get up and watch T.V. I watch Fraggle Rock with Pogo. A giant chases Pogo and gets him in a trap. I wrap up in my blanket and go to sleep on the couch.

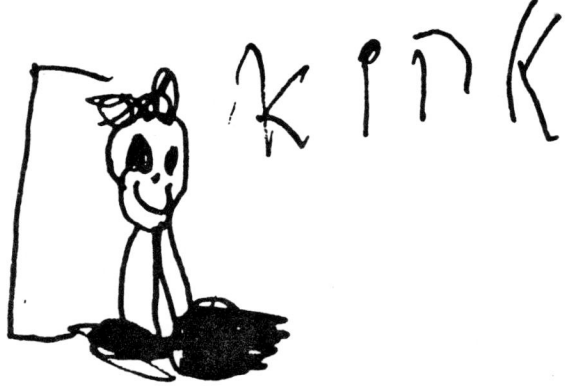

The next day mom takes me for an allergy shot. I wait in the waiting room until they say, "Kirk, come on in." They make me sit in a special room. The doctor or the nurse sticks a

Appendix A 111

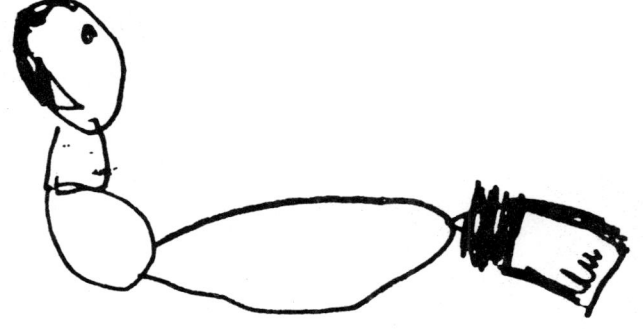

needle in my arm. It feels like a big knife is going in my arm. I never cry but hold my legs out straight and stiff and curl my toes. They put a Snoopy band-aid on my arm and then they give me a sucker and gum.

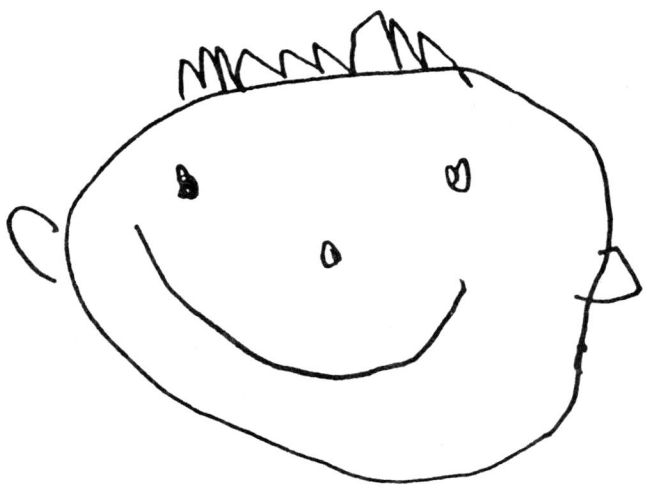

This year I am going to see Dr. Robertson, my new doctor. He will put me on a new diet, fruit, honey and vinegar. I won't have to take shots or blood tests anymore.

Appendix B
The Allergy Kid, Part II

The Allergy Kid Part II

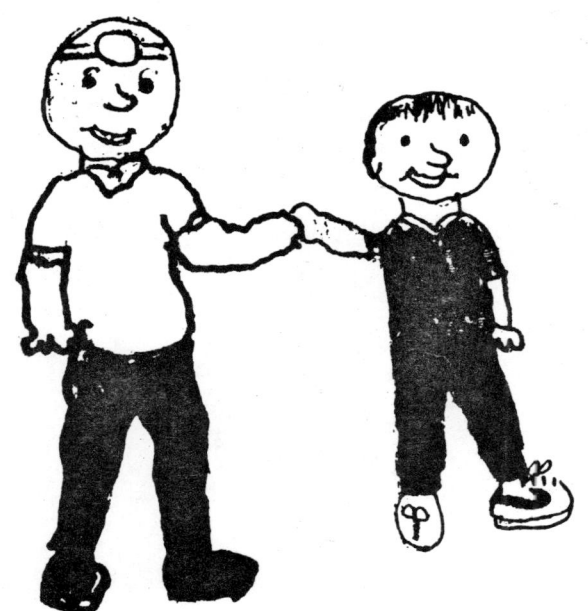

by
Kirk Boster

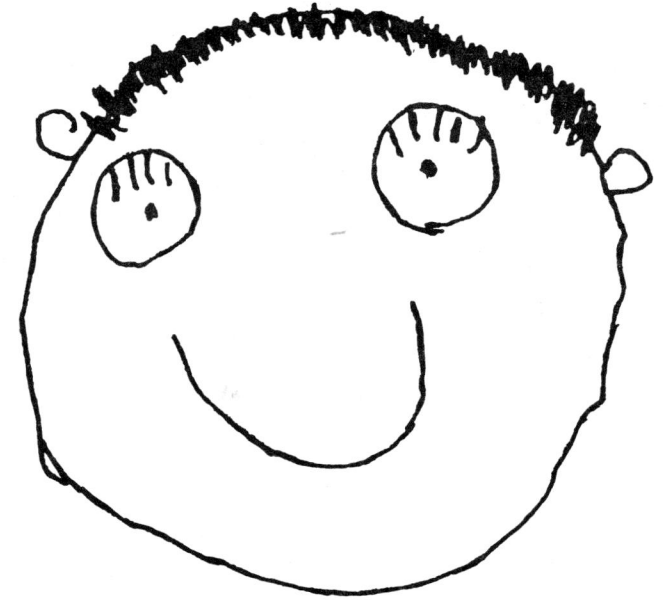

If you have asthma or allergies you should meet Dr. Robertson, He's my friend. He made me feel alot better.

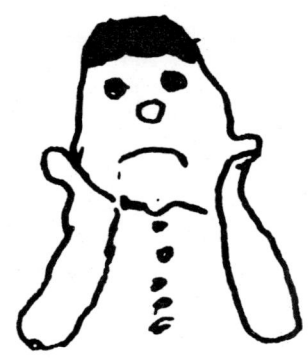

I was afraid to go see him. I was afraid of more shots and more blood tests. Having asthma is boring — getting sick and not being able to breathe — is not very fun.

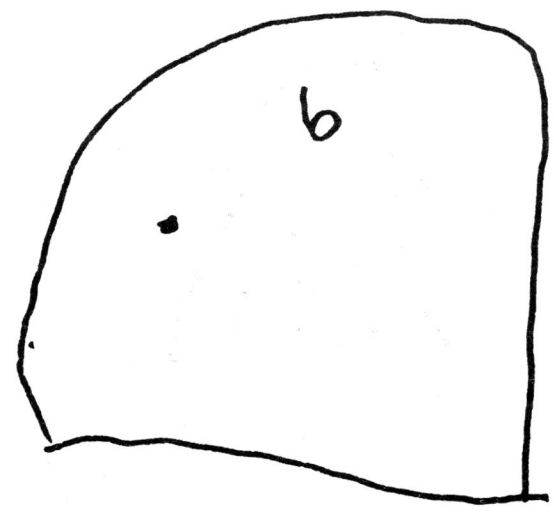

Dr. Robertson wasn't scary after I got use to his treatments. After you sit in the waiting room the Betty nurse calls you back to room six and the doctor is ready to meet you.

Appendix B

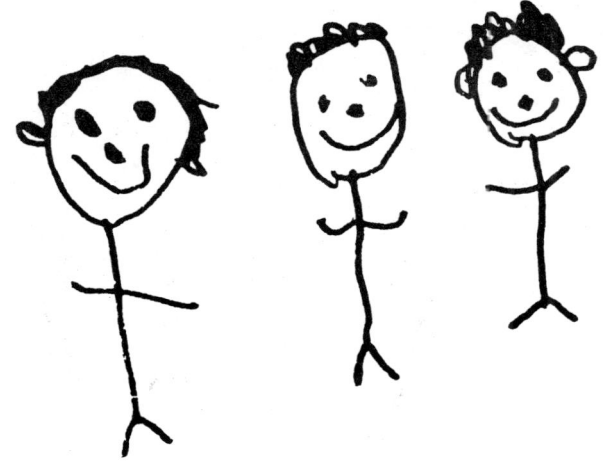

Your Mom and Dad get to go to.
He told me he wouldn't hurt
anyone but the devil. Then he
showed me the suction machine.
I said "what does that do?" He
said it helps suck the mucous out of

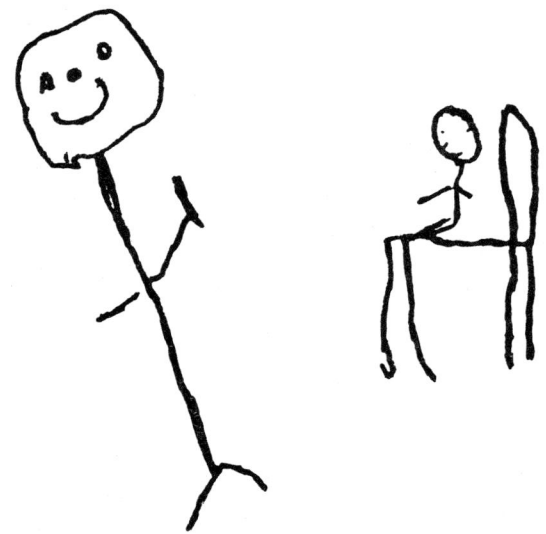

your system. "What is mucous?"
"Snot is what you call it." Then
he puts a screwdriver up my nose
to open it up and suck more mucous
out.

Appendix B

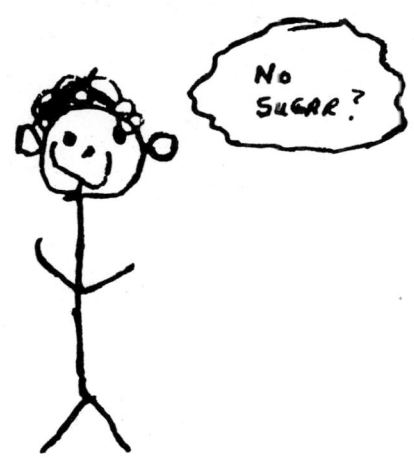

He told me that sugar is poisonous and it makes people sick. Don't eat preservatives! Drink honey and vinegar, and eat lots of fresh fruits and vegetables.

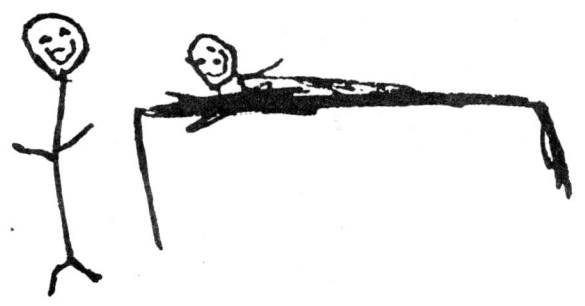

Dr. Robertson had me lay down and put his hands on my back and slides them up and down. Sometimes he sticks his pointy finger down my throat. Then I have to go down and tell Leoma to give me a colonic.

 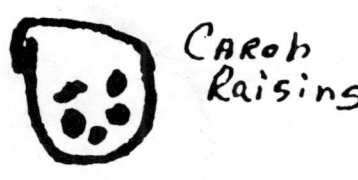

"I don't want to talk about colonies!"
When you get hungry you can go to the health food store and get fruit leather or carob raisins, they have a lot of good stuff.

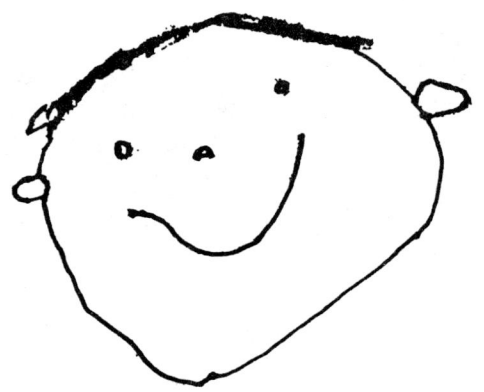

I feel lots better now and don't have much trouble breathing. I don't take medicine just supplements. I feel sad because I can't have candy and cookies like my friends, but someday I will have big muscles.
Thank you Dr. Robertson!!